TABLE OF CONTENTS

DISCLAIMER

The information provided in "A Woman's Guide to Nutrition: Fueling Your Body with the Right Foods for Every Stage of Life" is for educational and informational purposes only. It is not intended as a substitute for professional medical advice, diagnosis, or treatment. Always seek the advice of your physician or other qualified health provider with any questions you may have regarding a medical condition or before starting any new diet or exercise program.

The author and publisher disclaim any liability arising directly or indirectly from the use of this book. The reader assumes full responsibility for any actions taken based on the information contained herein.

Every effort has been made to ensure that the information in this book is accurate and up-to-date. However, the author and publisher make no guarantees about the completeness, reliability, and accuracy of the content. Any reliance you place on such information is therefore strictly at your own risk.

A WOMAN'S GUIDE TO NUTRITION

Fueling your body with the right foods for every stage of life

CLARISSA AUSTIN

INTRODUCTION

THE IMPORTANCE OF NUTRITION FOR WOMEN
Nutrition is the cornerstone of health and well-being, playing a crucial role in every aspect of our lives. For women, the significance of proper nutrition is even more profound, as it not only affects individual health but also impacts family and community wellness. Women's nutritional needs are unique and evolve through different life stages, from childhood and adolescence to adulthood, pregnancy, and menopause. Understanding and addressing these needs is essential for fostering a healthy, vibrant life.

THE ROLE OF NUTRITION IN WOMEN'S HEALTH
Proper nutrition provides the essential building blocks for the body's growth, repair, and maintenance. For women, these needs are particularly dynamic due to physiological changes, hormonal fluctuations, and the demands of pregnancy and breastfeeding. A well-balanced diet can help prevent chronic diseases such as heart disease, diabetes, and osteoporosis, which disproportionately affect women. Moreover, good nutrition is integral to maintaining a healthy weight, supporting mental health, and ensuring overall physical well-being.

Supporting Hormonal Balance and Reproductive Health

Hormonal balance is critical for women's health, influencing everything from mood and energy levels to reproductive health. Nutrients like omega-3 fatty acids, B vitamins, and magnesium play key roles in supporting hormonal functions and alleviating symptoms of hormonal imbalances, such as those experienced during premenstrual syndrome (PMS), pregnancy, and menopause. Proper nutrition can help mitigate the discomfort of these natural phases, enhancing quality of life.

Nutrition During Pregnancy and Lactation

Pregnancy and lactation are periods of increased nutritional demands, as a woman's body supports the growth and development of her baby. Adequate intake of key nutrients, such as folic acid, iron, calcium, and DHA, is crucial for preventing birth defects, promoting healthy fetal development, and ensuring maternal health. Breastfeeding mothers also need to maintain a nutrient-rich diet to support milk production and their own recovery postpartum.

Promoting Mental and Emotional Well-being

The connection between diet and mental health is increasingly recognized. Nutrient-dense foods can help stabilize mood, reduce stress, and improve cognitive function. For women, who are statistically more likely to experience depression and anxiety, nutrition can be a powerful tool for mental and emotional resilience. Foods rich in antioxidants, healthy fats, and essential vitamins and minerals support brain health and emotional stability.

Preventing and Managing Chronic Conditions

Chronic conditions such as osteoporosis, cardiovascular disease, and certain cancers are prevalent among women. A diet rich in fruits, vegetables, whole grains, lean proteins, and healthy fats can help prevent these conditions by reducing inflammation, supporting immune function, and promoting cardiovascular health. Additionally, managing conditions like polycystic ovary syndrome (PCOS) and endometriosis can be significantly improved through tailored nutritional strategies.

Empowering Women Through Nutrition Education

Knowledge is power, and understanding the fundamentals of nutrition empowers women to make informed choices about their health. This book aims to provide comprehensive, evidence-based information on nutrition tailored specifically to women's needs. By equipping women with the tools and knowledge to nourish their bodies effectively, we can foster a generation of healthier, more vibrant women.

CONCLUSION
Nutrition is not just about eating; it's about making choices that enhance our health and well-being throughout every stage of life. For women, good nutrition is a powerful ally in achieving a balanced, healthy life. As you embark on this journey through "A woman's Guide to Nutrition: Fueling Your Body with the Right Foods for Every Stage of Life," you'll discover the essential role that nutrition plays in supporting your health and happiness. Together, we will explore practical tips, delicious recipes, and the latest scientific insights to help you thrive at every age.

HOW TO USE THIS BOOK

Welcome to "A woman's Guide to Nutrition: Fueling Your Body with the Right Foods for Every Stage of Life." This book is designed to be your comprehensive resource for understanding and implementing the principles of good nutrition tailored specifically to women's unique needs. Whether you are a young adult, a mother-to-be, or navigating the changes of menopause, this guide will provide you with the knowledge and tools to make informed dietary choices that enhance your health and well-being.

NAVIGATING THE BOOK

This book is organized into six main parts, each focusing on different aspects of woman's nutrition:
The Basics of Woman's Nutrition: This section provides a foundation in nutrition science, covering essential nutrients, hydration, and the basics of a balanced diet.

Nutrition Across the Life Stages: Here, you'll find detailed information on the nutritional needs specific to various life stages, from adolescence to menopause and beyond.

Special Considerations: This part addresses unique dietary concerns, such as managing food allergies, optimizing nutrition for athletic performance, and understanding plant-based diets.

Practical Tips and Strategies: This section offers practical advice on meal planning, reading food labels, dining out, and considering supplements to ensure you can apply nutritional principles in your everyday life.

Recipes and Meal Plans: To help you put theory into practice, this part includes a variety of recipes and meal plans designed to meet your nutritional needs at every stage of life.

Moving Forward: The final section focuses on developing a healthy relationship with food, mindful eating, and strategies for maintaining motivation and overcoming challenges.

USING THE BOOK AS A REFERENCE

While this book is structured to be read from beginning to end, it is also designed to be a useful reference guide. Feel free to jump to sections that are most relevant to your current life stage or nutritional interests. Each chapter is self-contained, providing comprehensive information on its specific topic.

INCORPORATING NUTRITION INTO YOUR DAILY LIFE
Throughout the book, you'll find practical tips, real-life examples, and actionable advice to help you incorporate nutritional principles into your daily routine. Key takeaways and summaries at the end of each chapter will highlight the most important points, making it easier to remember and apply what you've learned.

RECIPES AND MEAL PLANS
The recipes and meal plans provided in Part V are designed to be simple, nutritious, and delicious. They are tailored to meet the unique needs of women at different stages of life and are easy to follow, even for those with a busy schedule. These recipes aim to inspire you to enjoy cooking and eating healthy foods that fuel your body and support your overall health.

INTERACTIVE ELEMENTS
To enhance your learning experience, this book includes various interactive elements:
Self-Assessment Quizzes: These will help you evaluate your current nutritional knowledge and identify areas for improvement.

Checklists and Worksheets: Practical tools to assist you in meal planning, grocery shopping, and tracking your nutritional intake.

Real-Life Case Studies: Inspirational stories from women who have successfully improved their health through nutrition.

CONCLUSION
"A woman's Guide to Nutrition" is more than just a book; it's a lifelong companion on your journey to better health. By understanding and implementing the nutritional principles outlined here, you will be empowered to make choices that enhance your well-being at every stage of life. Use this book as your guide to navigating the complex world of nutrition with confidence and ease. Here's to a healthier, happier you!

THE BASICS OF WOMEN'S NUTRITION

UNDERSTANDING MACRONUTRIENTS: CARBOHYDRATES, PROTEINS, AND FATS
Macronutrients—carbohydrates, proteins, and fats—are the primary nutrients our bodies need in large amounts to function properly. Each macronutrient plays a unique role in maintaining our health and well-being. Understanding how these macronutrients work and how to incorporate them into your diet is essential for achieving optimal health. This chapter will delve into the basics of carbohydrates, proteins, and fats, their functions, and how to make healthy choices.

CARBOHYDRATES: THE BODY'S PRIMARY ENERGY SOURCE
Carbohydrates are the body's main source of energy. They are found in foods such as fruits, vegetables, grains, and legumes. Carbohydrates are classified into two main types: simple and complex.

Simple Carbohydrates: These are sugars found in fruits, milk, and sweeteners like honey and table sugar. While they provide quick energy, they can also lead to rapid spikes and crashes in blood sugar levels.

Complex Carbohydrates: These include starches and fiber found in whole grains, legumes, and vegetables. They provide sustained energy and are essential for digestive health due to their fiber content.

WHY CARBOHYDRATES ARE IMPORTANT:
Energy Production: Carbohydrates are broken down into glucose, which is the primary fuel for our cells, especially during high-intensity activities.
Brain Function: The brain relies heavily on glucose for energy, making carbohydrates crucial for cognitive functions.

Digestive Health: Fiber, a type of carbohydrate, promotes healthy digestion and can prevent constipation.

HEALTHY CARBOHYDRATE CHOICES:
Opt for whole grains like brown rice, quinoa, and whole wheat bread.
Include a variety of fruits and vegetables in your diet.
Limit intake of refined sugars and processed foods.

PROTEINS: THE BUILDING BLOCKS OF THE BODY
Proteins are essential for building and repairing tissues, making enzymes and hormones, and supporting immune function. They are composed of amino acids, which are the building blocks of proteins.

Complete Proteins: These contain all nine essential amino acids that the body cannot produce on its own. Animal products like meat, dairy, and eggs are complete proteins.

Incomplete Proteins: These lack one or more essential amino acids and are found in plant-based sources like beans, nuts, and grains. Combining different plant-based proteins can provide all essential amino acids.

WHY PROTEINS ARE IMPORTANT:
Muscle Repair and Growth: Protein is crucial for repairing and building muscle tissues, especially after exercise.

Enzyme and Hormone Production: Proteins are vital for producing enzymes that aid in digestion and hormones that regulate body functions.
Immune Support: Antibodies, which help fight infections, are proteins.

HEALTHY PROTEIN CHOICES:
Include lean meats like chicken, turkey, and fish.
Incorporate plant-based proteins such as beans, lentils, tofu, and nuts.
Choose low-fat dairy products.

FATS: ESSENTIAL FOR HEALTH
Fats are essential for absorbing fat-soluble vitamins (A, D, E, and K), providing energy, and supporting cell growth. There are several types of fats, each with different effects on health.

Saturated Fats: Found in animal products and some plant oils, these fats can raise LDL (bad) cholesterol levels. Limit intake of saturated fats to support heart health.

Unsaturated Fats: These are healthier fats found in olive oil, avocados, nuts, and seeds. They help reduce LDL cholesterol and are beneficial for heart health.

Trans Fats: Found in some processed and fried foods, trans fats should be avoided as they can increase the risk of heart disease.

WHY FATS ARE IMPORTANT:
Energy Storage: Fats provide a concentrated source of energy and are stored for future use.
Nutrient Absorption: Fats help absorb essential fat-soluble vitamins.
Cell Structure: Fats are a key component of cell membranes and help maintain their integrity.

HEALTHY FAT CHOICES:
Use olive oil or avocado oil for cooking.
Include fatty fish like salmon and mackerel in your diet.
Eat nuts, seeds, and avocados as healthy fat sources.

BALANCING MACRONUTRIENTS

Achieving a balanced intake of carbohydrates, proteins, and fats is crucial for overall health. The proportion of each macronutrient may vary depending on individual health goals, activity levels, and life stages.

HERE ARE SOME GENERAL GUIDELINES:
Carbohydrates: Aim for 45-65% of your daily calories from carbohydrates, focusing on whole grains, fruits, and vegetables.

Proteins: Ensure 10-35% of your daily calories come from protein sources, including both animal and plant-based options.

Fats: 20-35% of your daily calories should come from fats, with an emphasis on unsaturated fats.
By understanding and balancing these macronutrients, you can create a diet that supports your energy needs, maintains your health, and helps prevent chronic diseases. Use this knowledge to make informed dietary choices that fit your lifestyle and health goals.

THE ROLE OF MICRONUTRIENTS: VITAMINS AND MINERALS
Micronutrients, which include vitamins and minerals, are essential for maintaining health and preventing disease. Unlike macronutrients (carbohydrates, proteins, and fats), which are needed in large quantities, micronutrients are required in smaller amounts. However, their impact on health is significant. This chapter explores the vital roles that vitamins and minerals play in the body, the consequences of deficiencies, and how to ensure you get an adequate intake through diet.

UNDERSTANDING VITAMINS
Vitamins are organic compounds that the body needs to function properly. They are classified into two categories: water-soluble and fat-soluble.

Water-Soluble Vitamins: These vitamins dissolve in water and are not stored in the body, meaning they need to be consumed regularly. They include the B-complex vitamins and vitamin C.
B-Complex Vitamins: These include B1 (thiamine), B2 (riboflavin), B3 (niacin), B5 (pantothenic acid), B6 (pyridoxine), B7 (biotin), B9 (folate), and B12 (cobalamin). They are essential for energy production, brain function, and cell metabolism.

Vitamin C: Important for the growth and repair of tissues, vitamin C is also a powerful antioxidant that helps protect cells from damage and supports the immune system.

Fat-Soluble Vitamins: These vitamins are absorbed along with fats in the diet and can be stored in the body's fatty tissues and liver. They include vitamins A, D, E, and K.
Vitamin A: Crucial for vision, immune function, and skin health.

Vitamin D: Important for bone health as it helps the body absorb calcium. It also supports immune function.
Vitamin E: Acts as an antioxidant, protecting cells from damage, and supports immune function.
Vitamin K: Essential for blood clotting and bone health.

UNDERSTANDING MINERALS
Minerals are inorganic elements that play a key role in a wide range of bodily functions. They are categorized as major minerals and trace minerals based on the amounts needed by the body.

Major Minerals: These are needed in larger amounts and include calcium, phosphorus, potassium, sodium, magnesium, sulfur, and chloride.

Calcium: Vital for bone and teeth health, muscle function, and nerve signaling.

Phosphorus: Important for the formation of bones and teeth, and involved in energy production. Helps regulate fluid balance, muscle contractions, and nerve signals.

Sodium: Essential for maintaining fluid balance and nerve function.

Magnesium: Involved in over 300 enzymatic reactions, including energy production, muscle function, and bone health.

Trace Minerals: These are needed in smaller amounts and include iron, zinc, iodine, selenium, copper, manganese, fluoride, chromium, and molybdenum.

Iron: Crucial for the formation of hemoglobin, which carries oxygen in the blood.
Zinc: Important for immune function, wound healing, and DNA synthesis.
Iodine: Essential for thyroid function, which regulates metabolism.
Selenium: Acts as an antioxidant and supports thyroid function.

THE IMPORTANCE OF MICRONUTRIENTS
Micronutrients are involved in virtually every process in the body. Here are some of their key roles:
Energy Production: B-vitamins are coenzymes in energy metabolism, helping convert food into energy.

Immune Function: Vitamins A, C, D, and E, as well as minerals like zinc and selenium, support a healthy immune system.

Bone Health: Calcium, phosphorus, magnesium, vitamin D, and vitamin K are crucial for maintaining strong bones and preventing osteoporosis.

Antioxidant Defense: Vitamins C and E, along with selenium and zinc, help protect cells from oxidative stress and damage.

Blood Health: Iron is necessary for producing hemoglobin, while vitamin K is essential for blood clotting.

CONSEQUENCES OF MICRONUTRIENT DEFICIENCIES
Micronutrient deficiencies can lead to a range of health problems, including:

Anemia: Caused by a lack of iron, vitamin B12, or folate, leading to fatigue and weakness.
Scurvy: Resulting from vitamin C deficiency, characterized by bleeding gums and weakened immune function.
Rickets and Osteoporosis: Due to vitamin D deficiency, leading to weakened bones.
Night Blindness: Caused by a lack of vitamin A, affecting vision.
Impaired Immune Function: Due to deficiencies in various vitamins and minerals, increasing susceptibility to infections.

ENSURING ADEQUATE INTAKE
To ensure you get enough vitamins and minerals, focus on a balanced and varied diet. Here are some tips:
Eat a Rainbow: Include a variety of colorful fruits and vegetables to get a wide range of vitamins and antioxidants.
Choose Whole Grains: Whole grains are rich in B-vitamins and trace minerals.
Include Dairy or Fortified Alternatives: For calcium, vitamin D, and other essential nutrients.
Incorporate Lean Proteins: Such as meat, fish, beans, and legumes, which provide iron, zinc, and other minerals.
Consider Supplements: If you have dietary restrictions or specific health conditions, supplements may be necessary, but consult with a healthcare provider first.

CONCLUSION
Micronutrients, though needed in small amounts, are vital for overall health and well-being. By understanding the roles of vitamins and minerals and ensuring a balanced diet, you can support your body's complex functions and maintain optimal health. Use this knowledge to make informed dietary choices that meet your nutritional needs and enhance your quality of life.

HYDRATION: THE ESSENTIAL ELEMENT
Hydration is a fundamental aspect of nutrition that is often overlooked. Water is essential for nearly every function in the human body, from regulating temperature to facilitating digestion and maintaining cellular health. Understanding the importance of proper hydration and how to maintain it can significantly enhance overall health and well-being. This chapter delves into the critical role of water in the body, the signs of dehydration, and practical tips for staying hydrated.

THE ROLE OF WATER IN THE BODY
Water makes up about 60% of an adult human body and is involved in numerous physiological processes:

Regulating Body Temperature: Through sweating and respiration, water helps maintain a stable body temperature.

Transporting Nutrients and Oxygen: Water is a key component of blood, which delivers essential nutrients and oxygen to cells.

Removing Waste: Water aids in the excretion of waste products through urine, sweat, and feces.

Digestive Health: Water is essential for the digestion and absorption of food, as well as the prevention of constipation.

Joint Lubrication: Synovial fluid, which lubricates and cushions joints, is primarily composed of water.

Protecting Tissues and Organs: Water helps cushion and protect vital organs and tissues.

SIGNS OF DEHYDRATION
Dehydration occurs when the body loses more water than it takes in, leading to a deficit. It can impair physical and cognitive functions and, in severe cases, can be life-threatening. Common signs of dehydration include:

Thirst: The body's natural response to needing more fluids.

Dry Mouth and Skin: A lack of moisture can cause dryness.

Dark Urine: Urine should be light yellow; darker urine indicates concentrated waste and a need for more water.

Fatigue: Dehydration can lead to decreased energy levels and feelings of tiredness.

Headaches: Lack of adequate hydration can cause headaches and migraines.

Dizziness and Confusion: Severe dehydration can affect cognitive function and lead to disorientation.

Muscle Cramps: Dehydration can cause muscles to contract involuntarily.

DAILY WATER NEEDS

Individual water needs can vary based on factors such as age, weight, climate, physical activity, and overall health. However, general guidelines can help ensure adequate hydration:

Men: Approximately 3.7 liters (about 13 cups) of total water intake per day.

Women: Approximately 2.7 liters (about 9 cups) of total water intake per day.
These recommendations include all fluids consumed, not just water, and also consider the water content in foods.

FACTORS AFFECTING HYDRATION
Several factors can influence your hydration needs:

Physical Activity: Exercise increases water loss through sweat, requiring higher fluid intake.
Climate: Hot and humid weather increases sweating, necessitating more water.
Health Conditions: Illnesses such as fever, vomiting, and diarrhea can lead to increased fluid loss.
Pregnancy and Breastfeeding: These stages increase water needs to support the growing fetus and milk production.

PRACTICAL TIPS FOR STAYING HYDRATED
Maintaining proper hydration is straightforward with some practical strategies:

Carry a Water Bottle: Keep a reusable water bottle with you to encourage regular drinking.
Set Reminders: Use phone alarms or apps to remind you to drink water throughout the day.

Infuse Water with Flavor: Add slices of fruits, vegetables, or herbs to your water for a refreshing twist.

Eat Water-Rich Foods: Include fruits and vegetables with high water content, such as cucumbers, watermelon, and oranges, in your diet.
Monitor Your Urine: Use the color of your urine as a guide; aim for light yellow.

Drink Before You're Thirsty: Thirst is a late indicator of dehydration, so drink fluids regularly.

HYDRATION AND EXERCISE
For those who engage in regular physical activity, hydration becomes even more critical:

Before Exercise: Drink about 500 ml (17 ounces) of water 2-3 hours before exercise.

During Exercise: Drink about 200-300 ml (7-10 ounces) every 20 minutes during exercise, adjusting for intensity and climate.

After Exercise: Replenish fluids lost through sweat by drinking water or an electrolyte solution.

HYDRATION MYTHS
There are many myths surrounding hydration. Here are a few clarifications:

Myth: You need exactly 8 glasses of water a day: Individual needs vary, and total fluid intake includes all beverages and food.

Myth: Coffee and tea dehydrate you: While they have a mild diuretic effect, they still contribute to your overall fluid intake.

Myth: Clear urine is the goal: Light yellow urine indicates proper hydration, not clear.

CONCLUSION
Hydration is a vital component of health that supports countless bodily functions. By understanding your individual hydration needs and incorporating simple habits into your daily routine, you can ensure that you stay properly hydrated. Remember, water is essential for life, and maintaining adequate hydration is a fundamental step toward achieving and maintaining overall well-being.

BUILDING A BALANCED PLATE: PORTION SIZES AND FOOD GROUPS
Creating a balanced plate is a cornerstone of healthy eating. A balanced plate ensures that you get the right mix of nutrients from various food groups in appropriate portion sizes. This chapter will guide you through understanding the major food groups, the importance of portion sizes, and practical tips for building a balanced plate that meets your nutritional needs.

UNDERSTANDING THE MAJOR FOOD GROUPS
A balanced diet includes a variety of foods from the following five major food groups:
Vegetables
Fruits
Grains
Protein Foods
Dairy
Each food group provides essential nutrients that are crucial for maintaining health and preventing chronic diseases.

1. Vegetables:
Vegetables are rich in vitamins, minerals, fiber, and antioxidants. They should form a significant portion of your plate.

Types of Vegetables: Dark leafy greens, red and orange vegetables, starchy vegetables, and legumes (beans and peas).

Recommended Intake: Aim for at least 2.5 cups of vegetables per day.

2. Fruits:

Fruits are excellent sources of essential vitamins, minerals, and fiber. They also provide natural sugars for energy.

Types of Fruits: Berries, citrus fruits, melons, and stone fruits.
Recommended Intake: Aim for at least 1.5-2 cups of fruit per day.

3. Grains:

Grains are a major source of energy and provide essential nutrients such as fiber, B vitamins, and minerals.

Types of Grains: Whole grains (brown rice, quinoa, oats) and refined grains (white bread, white rice).

Recommended Intake: At least half of your grain intake should be whole grains. Aim for 6-8 servings per day, with one serving being equivalent to one slice of bread or half a cup of cooked grains.

4. Protein Foods:

Protein is essential for building and repairing tissues, and it also plays a role in immune function and hormone production.

Types of Protein: Lean meats, poultry, fish, beans, peas, lentils, nuts, seeds, and soy products.

Recommended Intake: Aim for 5-6.5 ounces of protein foods per day.

5. Dairy:

Dairy products are rich in calcium, vitamin D, and other essential nutrients important for bone health.

Types of Dairy: Milk, yogurt, cheese, and fortified plant-based alternatives.

Recommended Intake: Aim for 3 cups of dairy per day.

IMPORTANCE OF PORTION SIZES
Understanding portion sizes is key to maintaining a balanced diet and avoiding overeating or undernourishment. Portion control helps ensure you get the right amount of nutrients without consuming excess calories.

TIPS FOR MANAGING PORTION SIZES:

Use Smaller Plates and Bowls: This can help you eat smaller portions and feel satisfied.

Read Nutrition Labels: Pay attention to serving sizes on food labels to understand how much you're eating.

Measure Your Food: Use measuring cups and spoons to serve appropriate portions, especially for high-calorie foods.

Mindful Eating: Eat slowly and pay attention to your hunger and fullness cues to avoid overeating.

BUILDING A BALANCED PLATE
To create a balanced plate, aim to include a variety of foods from different food groups in each meal. Here's a simple guide to follow:

1. Fill Half Your Plate with Vegetables and Fruits:

Aim for a variety of colors and types to maximize nutrient intake.
Vegetables can be cooked or raw, and fruits can be fresh, frozen, or canned (in water or natural juice).

2. Fill a Quarter of Your Plate with Lean Protein:

Include a variety of protein sources such as poultry, fish, beans, lentils, tofu, and nuts.
Choose lean cuts of meat and remove visible fat before cooking.

3. Fill a Quarter of Your Plate with Whole Grains:
Opt for whole grains like brown rice, quinoa, whole wheat pasta, and oats.
Avoid refined grains and choose whole grain versions of bread, cereals, and pasta.

4. Include a Serving of Dairy or Dairy Alternatives:

Add a serving of low-fat or fat-free milk, yogurt, or cheese.
For non-dairy options, choose fortified plant-based milk and yogurt.

PRACTICAL TIPS FOR A BALANCED DIET

Plan Your Meals: Plan your meals and snacks ahead of time to ensure they are balanced and include a variety of food groups.

Stay Hydrated: Drink plenty of water throughout the day. Limit sugary drinks and opt for water, herbal teas, or other low-calorie beverages.

Cook at Home: Preparing meals at home allows you to control ingredients and portion sizes, ensuring healthier choices.

Mindful Eating: Focus on your food, savor each bite, and avoid distractions like TV or smartphones while eating.

Snack Wisely: Choose healthy snacks such as fruits, vegetables, nuts, and yogurt to keep your energy levels stable throughout the day.

CONCLUSION
Building a balanced plate is a practical approach to ensuring you get the right mix of nutrients from different food groups. By paying attention to portion sizes and including a variety of foods in your diet, you can support your overall health and well-being. Use this guide to make informed choices and create balanced, nutritious meals that meet your individual needs.

NUTRITION ACROSS THE LIFE STAGES

CHILDHOOD AND ADOLESCENCE: BUILDING A STRONG FOUNDATION
Childhood and adolescence are critical periods for growth and development. Proper nutrition during these stages is essential for building a strong foundation for lifelong health. This chapter will explore the unique nutritional needs of children and adolescents, the importance of healthy eating habits, and practical strategies for supporting optimal growth and development.

NUTRITIONAL NEEDS IN CHILDHOOD
During childhood, the body undergoes rapid growth and development, requiring a variety of nutrients to support this process. Key nutritional needs include:

1. Calories: Children need adequate calories to fuel their growing bodies. Caloric needs vary based on age, sex, and activity level.

Toddlers (1-3 years): Approximately 1,000-1,400 calories per day.
Preschoolers (4-6 years): Approximately 1,200-1,800 calories per day.
School-age children (7-12 years): Approximately 1,600-2,400 calories per day.

2. Protein: Essential for growth, muscle development, and immune function.

Recommended Intake: 13-19 grams per day for young children and 34-52 grams per day for older children, depending on age and sex.

3. Carbohydrates: The primary source of energy, especially important for active children.

Recommended Intake: 45-65% of daily calories.

4. Fats: Necessary for brain development, hormone production, and absorption of fat-soluble vitamins.

Recommended Intake: 25-35% of daily calories for children ages 4-18 years.

5. Vitamins and Minerals: Vital for various bodily functions, including bone growth, immune support, and cognitive development. Key nutrients include:

Calcium: Important for bone health. Recommended intake: 700-1,300 mg per day.
Iron: Essential for blood health. Recommended intake: 7-15 mg per day.
Vitamin D: Supports bone health and immune function. Recommended intake: 600 IU per day.

NUTRITIONAL NEEDS IN ADOLESCENCE
Adolescence is marked by rapid growth spurts, hormonal changes, and increased physical activity, leading to higher nutritional needs. Important considerations include:

1. Increased Caloric Needs: Adolescents require more calories to support growth and increased activity levels.

Teenage boys: Approximately 2,200-3,200 calories per day.
Teenage girls: Approximately 1,800-2,400 calories per day.

2. Protein: Continues to be important for growth, muscle development, and repair.

Recommended Intake: 46-52 grams per day for girls and 52-66 grams per day for boys.

3. Calcium and Vitamin D: Crucial for achieving peak bone mass and preventing future osteoporosis.

Calcium: 1,300 mg per day.
Vitamin D: 600-1,000 IU per day.

4. Iron: Increased need, especially for menstruating girls.

Recommended Intake: 11-15 mg per day.

5. Folic Acid: Important for cell growth and development, particularly for girls of childbearing age.

Recommended Intake: 400 mcg per day.

IMPORTANCE OF HEALTHY EATING HABITS
Establishing healthy eating habits during childhood and adolescence sets the stage for lifelong health. Key aspects include:

1. Balanced Diet: Ensure a varied diet that includes all food groups: fruits, vegetables, grains, protein foods, and dairy.

2. Regular Meals and Snacks: Encourage regular meals and healthy snacks to maintain energy levels and support growth.

3. Limiting Sugary and Processed Foods: Reduce intake of sugary drinks, snacks, and highly processed foods to prevent obesity and related health issues.

4. Hydration: Promote drinking plenty of water and limiting sugary beverages.

5. Family Meals: Eating together as a family can promote healthy eating habits and provide an opportunity to model good nutrition.

PRACTICAL STRATEGIES FOR SUPPORTING GROWTH AND DEVELOPMENT

1. Involve Children in Meal Planning and Preparation: This can encourage interest in healthy foods and teach valuable cooking skills.

2. Create a Positive Eating Environment: Avoid pressuring children to eat and make mealtimes pleasant and stress-free.

3. Educate on Nutrition: Teach children and adolescents about the importance of different nutrients and how to make healthy food choices.

4. Encourage Physical Activity: Combine good nutrition with regular physical activity to support overall health and development.

5. Monitor Growth and Development: Regular check-ups with healthcare providers can help ensure children and adolescents are growing and developing appropriately.

ADDRESSING COMMON CHALLENGES

1. Picky Eating: Encourage trying new foods without pressure. Offer a variety of foods and be patient.

2. Busy Schedules: Plan ahead for healthy meals and snacks. Use weekends to prepare meals for the week.

3. Peer Influence and Media: Teach children to critically evaluate food advertisements and make healthy choices despite peer pressure.

CONCLUSION
Proper nutrition during childhood and adolescence is crucial for building a strong foundation for lifelong health. By understanding the unique nutritional needs of these stages, promoting healthy eating habits, and implementing practical strategies, parents and caregivers can support optimal growth and development. Remember, the habits formed during these formative years can influence health outcomes well into adulthood.

NUTRITION FOR YOUNG ADULTS: ENERGY AND VITALITY
Young adulthood, typically defined as ages 18 to 30, is a dynamic phase marked by new responsibilities, increased independence, and significant lifestyle changes. Proper nutrition during this period is essential for sustaining energy, promoting mental clarity, and maintaining overall health. This chapter explores the nutritional needs of young adults, the importance of balanced eating for energy and vitality, and practical strategies for maintaining a healthy diet.
NUTRITIONAL NEEDS OF YOUNG ADULTS
Young adults require a diet that supports their active lifestyles, academic or career demands, and ongoing physical development. Key nutritional needs include:

1. Calories: Caloric needs vary based on age, sex, weight, height, and activity level. On average:

Men: Approximately 2,400-3,000 calories per day.
Women: Approximately 1,800-2,400 calories per day.

2. Protein: Essential for muscle maintenance, immune function, and overall cellular health.

Recommended Intake: 46 grams per day for women and 56 grams per day for men, but individual needs may be higher depending on physical activity levels.

3. Carbohydrates: The primary source of energy, especially for brain function and physical activity.

Recommended Intake: 45-65% of total daily calories.

4. Fats: Necessary for hormone production, brain health, and absorption of fat-soluble vitamins.

Recommended Intake: 20-35% of total daily calories, focusing on healthy fats like those from nuts, seeds, avocados, and fish.

5. Vitamins and Minerals: Crucial for various bodily functions, including:

Calcium and Vitamin D: Important for bone health. Aim for 1,000 mg of calcium and 600-800 IU of vitamin D per day.
Iron: Essential for oxygen transport and energy levels. Aim for 8 mg per day for men and 18 mg per day for women.
B Vitamins: Important for energy metabolism and brain function. Ensure adequate intake of B6, B12, and folic acid through diet or supplements.

IMPORTANCE OF BALANCED EATING FOR ENERGY AND VITALITY
A balanced diet not only supports physical health but also enhances mental and emotional well-being. Key components include:

1. Diverse Food Groups: Incorporate a variety of foods from all food groups to ensure a wide range of nutrients.

Fruits and Vegetables: Rich in vitamins, minerals, and antioxidants. Aim for at least 5 servings per day.
Whole Grains: Provide sustained energy and fiber. Choose whole grain bread, brown rice, quinoa, and oats.
Lean Proteins: Include sources such as chicken, fish, beans, lentils, and tofu.
Healthy Fats: Avocados, nuts, seeds, and olive oil are excellent sources of healthy fats.

Dairy or Alternatives: Ensure adequate intake of calcium and vitamin D through milk, yogurt, cheese, or fortified plant-based alternatives.

2. Regular Meals and Snacks: Eating regular meals and healthy snacks helps maintain energy levels throughout the day.

Breakfast: Start the day with a nutritious breakfast to boost metabolism and energy.
Balanced Snacks: Choose snacks that combine protein and fiber, such as yogurt with fruit, nuts with whole grain crackers, or hummus with veggies.

3. Hydration: Proper hydration is essential for energy, concentration, and overall health.

Water: Aim for at least 8 cups (2 liters) of water per day, more if physically active.
Limit Sugary Drinks: Avoid sugary sodas and energy drinks, which can lead to energy crashes.

PRACTICAL STRATEGIES FOR A HEALTHY DIET

1. Meal Planning and Preparation: Plan meals and snacks ahead of time to ensure balanced nutrition.

Batch Cooking: Prepare large portions of healthy meals and freeze them for later use.
Healthy Staples: Keep healthy staples like whole grains, lean proteins, and fresh produce on hand.

2. Smart Shopping: Make informed choices at the grocery store.

Shop the Perimeter: Focus on fresh produce, dairy, meat, and whole grains typically found around the store's perimeter.
Read Labels: Check nutrition labels for added sugars, unhealthy fats, and artificial ingredients.

3. Eating Out Wisely: Make healthier choices when dining out.

Portion Control: Be mindful of portion sizes, and consider sharing dishes or saving half for later.
Healthy Options: Choose restaurants that offer healthier options, and opt for grilled instead of fried foods, and salads or vegetables instead of fries.

4. Mindful Eating: Pay attention to hunger and fullness cues.

Avoid Distractions: Eat without distractions like TV or smartphones to better enjoy and regulate your food intake.
Slow Down: Take your time to eat, which can help prevent overeating and aid digestion.

ADDRESSING COMMON CHALLENGES

1. Busy Schedules: Manage a hectic lifestyle with quick, nutritious options.

Healthy On-the-Go: Keep portable snacks like nuts, fruit, and whole grain bars handy.
Prep Ahead: Prepare meals in advance to avoid relying on fast food or convenience items.

2. Budget Constraints: Eating healthy on a budget is possible with careful planning.

Bulk Buying: Purchase staples like grains, beans, and frozen vegetables in bulk.
Seasonal Produce: Buy fruits and vegetables in season for better prices and freshness.

3. Social Eating: Navigating social settings and peer pressure can be challenging.

Healthy Choices: Suggest restaurants with healthier options or bring a nutritious dish to gatherings.
Balance: Enjoy treats in moderation and balance indulgent meals with healthier choices.

CONCLUSION
Nutrition plays a vital role in maintaining energy, vitality, and overall health during young adulthood. By understanding your nutritional needs, making balanced food choices, and adopting practical strategies for healthy eating, you can support your active lifestyle and long-term well-being. Remember, the habits you establish now can positively influence your health for years to come.

PREGNANCY AND BREASTFEEDING: NUTRITIONAL NEEDS FOR MOTHER AND BABY
Pregnancy and breastfeeding are transformative periods in a woman's life, demanding increased nutritional support to ensure the health and development of both mother and baby. This chapter explores the essential nutrients needed during pregnancy and lactation, the importance of a balanced diet, and practical strategies for meeting these unique nutritional requirements.

NUTRITIONAL NEEDS DURING PREGNANCY
Pregnancy is a time of significant physiological changes, with increased demands for energy and nutrients to support fetal growth and development. Key nutrients include:

1. Folic Acid (Folate): Vital for preventing neural tube defects and supporting fetal brain development.
Recommended Intake: 600-800 mcg per day.

2. Iron: Essential for preventing maternal anemia and supporting fetal growth.

Recommended Intake: 27 mg per day.

3. Calcium and Vitamin D: Crucial for fetal bone development and maternal bone health.

Recommended Intake: Calcium - 1,000 mg per day; Vitamin D - 600 IU per day.

4. Omega-3 Fatty Acids: Support fetal brain and eye development.

Sources: Fatty fish (like salmon), walnuts, flaxseeds, and fortified foods.

5. Protein: Needed for maternal tissue growth and fetal development.

Recommended Intake: Additional 25 grams per day during pregnancy.

6. Zinc: Important for immune function and cell growth.

Recommended Intake: 11-13 mg per day.

7. Vitamins A, C, and B Vitamins: Essential for immune function, collagen formation, and overall health.

IMPORTANCE OF A BALANCED DIET DURING PREGNANCY
A balanced diet during pregnancy ensures that both mother and baby receive adequate nutrition. Focus on:

1. Fruits and Vegetables: Rich in vitamins, minerals, and fiber.

Variety: Aim for a colorful array to maximize nutrient intake.

2. Whole Grains: Provide energy and essential nutrients like folate and fiber.

Examples: Brown rice, whole wheat bread, quinoa.

3. Lean Proteins: Necessary for fetal growth and maternal tissue repair.

Sources: Lean meats, poultry, fish, beans, lentils, tofu.

4. Dairy or Dairy Alternatives: Important for calcium, vitamin D, and protein.

Options: Milk, yogurt, cheese, fortified plant-based alternatives.
5. Healthy Fats: Support fetal brain development and maternal health.

Sources: Avocados, nuts, seeds, olive oil, fatty fish.

NUTRITIONAL NEEDS DURING BREASTFEEDING

Breastfeeding continues to require increased nutritional support to promote milk production and sustain maternal health. Key nutrients include:

1. Fluids: Adequate hydration is crucial for milk production and maternal well-being.

Recommendation: Drink plenty of water throughout the day.

2. Calories: Additional energy is needed to support milk production and maternal recovery.

Recommendation: About 450-500 extra calories per day.

3. Omega-3 Fatty Acids: Support infant brain development through breast milk.

Sources: Fatty fish, flaxseeds, chia seeds.

4. Calcium and Vitamin D: Important for bone health, especially if maternal intake was inadequate during pregnancy.

Recommendation: Same as during pregnancy - Calcium 1,000 mg per day, Vitamin D 600 IU per day.

5. Protein: Supports milk production and maternal tissue repair.

Recommendation: Additional 25 grams per day during lactation.

PRACTICAL STRATEGIES FOR MEETING NUTRITIONAL NEEDS

1. Prenatal Supplements: Take a prenatal vitamin recommended by your healthcare provider to ensure adequate intake of essential nutrients.

2. Balanced Meals and Snacks: Plan meals that include a variety of food groups to meet nutrient needs throughout the day.

3. Hydration: Drink water regularly to support milk production and overall hydration.

4. Small, Frequent Meals: Eating smaller meals and snacks throughout the day can help manage energy levels and prevent hunger.

5. Listen to Your Body: Pay attention to hunger and fullness cues to guide eating patterns and ensure adequate nutrition.

ADDRESSING COMMON CONCERNS

1. Nausea and Food Aversions: If experiencing morning sickness or aversions to certain foods, focus on consuming small, frequent meals and snacks that are well-tolerated.

2. Vegetarian or Vegan Diets: Ensure adequate intake of essential nutrients like protein, iron, calcium, and vitamin B12 through fortified foods or supplements.

3. Consultation with Healthcare Provider: Discuss any specific dietary concerns or questions with your healthcare provider to ensure personalized guidance and support.

CONCLUSION

Nutrition plays a crucial role in supporting the health and well-being of both mother and baby during pregnancy and breastfeeding. By prioritizing a balanced diet rich in essential nutrients, staying hydrated, and seeking guidance from healthcare providers when needed, mothers can optimize their own health while providing the best possible start for their infants. Remember, each pregnancy and breastfeeding journey is unique, so listen to your body and make informed choices to support this transformative time in your life.

PREGNANCY AND BREASTFEEDING: NUTRITIONAL NEEDS FOR MOTHER AND BABY

Pregnancy and breastfeeding are transformative periods in a woman's life, demanding increased nutritional support to ensure the health and development of both mother and baby. This chapter explores the essential nutrients needed during pregnancy and lactation, the importance of a balanced diet, and practical strategies for meeting these unique nutritional requirements.

NUTRITIONAL NEEDS DURING PREGNANCY

Pregnancy is a time of significant physiological changes, with increased demands for energy and nutrients to support fetal growth and development. Key nutrients include:

1. Folic Acid (Folate): Vital for preventing neural tube defects and supporting fetal brain development.

Recommended Intake: 600-800 mcg per day.

2. Iron: Essential for preventing maternal anemia and supporting fetal growth.

Recommended Intake: 27 mg per day.

3. Calcium and Vitamin D: Crucial for fetal bone development and maternal bone health.

Recommended Intake: Calcium - 1,000 mg per day; Vitamin D - 600 IU per day.

4. Omega-3 Fatty Acids: Support fetal brain and eye development.

Sources: Fatty fish (like salmon), walnuts, flaxseeds, and fortified foods.

5. Protein: Needed for maternal tissue growth and fetal development.

Recommended Intake: Additional 25 grams per day during pregnancy.

6. Zinc: Important for immune function and cell growth.

Recommended Intake: 11-13 mg per day.

7. Vitamins A, C, and B Vitamins: Essential for immune function, collagen formation, and overall health.

IMPORTANCE OF A BALANCED DIET DURING PREGNANCY
A balanced diet during pregnancy ensures that both mother and baby receive adequate nutrition. Focus on:

1. Fruits and Vegetables: Rich in vitamins, minerals, and fiber.

Variety: Aim for a colorful array to maximize nutrient intake.

2. Whole Grains: Provide energy and essential nutrients like folate and fiber.

Examples: Brown rice, whole wheat bread, quinoa.

3. Lean Proteins: Necessary for fetal growth and maternal tissue repair.

Sources: Lean meats, poultry, fish, beans, lentils, tofu.

4. Dairy or Dairy Alternatives: Important for calcium, vitamin D, and protein.

Options: Milk, yogurt, cheese, fortified plant-based alternatives.

5. Healthy Fats: Support fetal brain development and maternal health.

Sources: Avocados, nuts, seeds, olive oil, fatty fish.

NUTRITIONAL NEEDS DURING BREASTFEEDING
Breastfeeding continues to require increased nutritional support to promote milk production and sustain maternal health. Key nutrients include:

1. Fluids: Adequate hydration is crucial for milk production and maternal well-being.

Recommendation: Drink plenty of water throughout the day.

2. Calories: Additional energy is needed to support milk production and maternal recovery.

Recommendation: About 450-500 extra calories per day.

3. Omega-3 Fatty Acids: Support infant brain development through breast milk.

Sources: Fatty fish, flaxseeds, chia seeds.

4. Calcium and Vitamin D: Important for bone health, especially if maternal intake was inadequate during pregnancy.

Recommendation: Same as during pregnancy - Calcium 1,000 mg per day, Vitamin D 600 IU per day.

5. Protein: Supports milk production and maternal tissue repair.

Recommendation: Additional 25 grams per day during lactation.

PRACTICAL STRATEGIES FOR MEETING NUTRITIONAL NEEDS

1. Prenatal Supplements: Take a prenatal vitamin recommended by your healthcare provider to ensure adequate intake of essential nutrients.

2. Balanced Meals and Snacks: Plan meals that include a variety of food groups to meet nutrient needs throughout the day.

3. Hydration: Drink water regularly to support milk production and overall hydration.

4. Small, Frequent Meals: Eating smaller meals and snacks throughout the day can help manage energy levels and prevent hunger.

5. Listen to Your Body: Pay attention to hunger and fullness cues to guide eating patterns and ensure adequate nutrition.

ADDRESSING COMMON CONCERNS

1. Nausea and Food Aversions: If experiencing morning sickness or aversions to certain foods, focus on consuming small, frequent meals and snacks that are well-tolerated.

2. Vegetarian or Vegan Diets: Ensure adequate intake of essential nutrients like protein, iron, calcium, and vitamin B12 through fortified foods or supplements.

3. Consultation with Healthcare Provider: Discuss any specific dietary concerns or questions with your healthcare provider to ensure personalized guidance and support.

CONCLUSION
Nutrition plays a crucial role in supporting the health and well-being of both mother and baby during pregnancy and breastfeeding. By prioritizing a balanced diet rich in essential nutrients, staying hydrated, and seeking guidance from healthcare providers when needed, mothers can optimize their own health while providing the best possible start for their infants. Remember, each pregnancy and breastfeeding journey is unique, so listen to your body and make informed choices to support this transformative time in your life.

MIDLIFE NUTRITION: BALANCING HORMONES AND METABOLISM
Midlife, typically spanning from ages 40 to 60, is characterized by various physiological changes, including hormonal fluctuations and changes in metabolism. Proper nutrition during this stage of life plays a crucial role in supporting overall health, managing weight, and mitigating age-related health risks. This chapter explores the nutritional needs of individuals during midlife, the impact of hormonal changes on metabolism, and practical strategies for maintaining optimal health and well-being.

NUTRITIONAL NEEDS DURING MIDLIFE
As individuals age, their nutritional needs evolve to support changes in metabolism, hormone levels, and overall health. Key considerations include:

1. Macronutrients:

Protein: Essential for maintaining muscle mass, which naturally declines with age. Aim for lean sources such as poultry, fish, beans, and tofu.
Carbohydrates: Choose complex carbohydrates like whole grains, fruits, vegetables, and legumes to support steady energy levels and fiber intake.
Healthy Fats: Include sources like nuts, seeds, avocados, and olive oil to support heart health and cognitive function.

2. Micronutrients:
Calcium and Vitamin D: Vital for bone health and reducing the risk of osteoporosis. Aim for 1,200 mg of calcium per day and 600-800 IU of vitamin D.
B Vitamins: Important for energy production and cognitive function. Include sources such as whole grains, leafy greens, and fortified cereals.
Omega-3 Fatty Acids: Support heart health and brain function. Include fatty fish (like salmon), flaxseeds, and walnuts in your diet.

3. Fiber: Essential for digestive health, managing cholesterol levels, and maintaining a healthy weight. Aim for at least 25 grams of fiber per day from whole grains, fruits, vegetables, and legumes.

4. Hydration: Maintain adequate hydration to support metabolism, cognitive function, and overall health. Aim for about 8 cups (2 liters) of water per day, adjusting based on activity level and climate.

HORMONAL CHANGES AND METABOLISM

During midlife, both men and women experience hormonal changes that can impact metabolism and overall health:

1. Menopause (Women): Declining estrogen levels can lead to changes in fat distribution, metabolism, and bone health.

Nutritional Focus: Support bone health with adequate calcium and vitamin D intake. Manage weight through balanced eating and regular physical activity.

2. Andropause (Men): Declining testosterone levels can affect muscle mass, energy levels, and overall vitality.

Nutritional Focus: Prioritize lean protein sources to support muscle maintenance and physical activity. Include zinc-rich foods like lean meats, shellfish, and legumes.

PRACTICAL STRATEGIES FOR MAINTAINING HEALTH

1. Balanced Diet: Emphasize whole foods, including fruits, vegetables, lean proteins, whole grains, and healthy fats.

Meal Planning: Plan meals ahead to ensure balanced nutrition and avoid reliance on processed foods.

2. Portion Control: Pay attention to portion sizes to manage calorie intake and support weight management.

3. Regular Physical Activity: Incorporate aerobic exercise, strength training, and flexibility exercises to support metabolism, muscle mass, and overall health.

4. Stress Management: Practice stress-reducing techniques such as meditation, yoga, or deep breathing exercises to support hormonal balance and overall well-being.

5. Regular Health Screenings: Schedule regular check-ups with healthcare providers to monitor blood pressure, cholesterol levels, bone density, and other health markers.

ADDRESSING COMMON HEALTH CONCERNS

1. Heart Health: Prioritize heart-healthy fats, limit saturated and trans fats, and monitor blood pressure and cholesterol levels.

2. Bone Health: Ensure adequate calcium and vitamin D intake to support bone density and reduce the risk of osteoporosis.

3. Cognitive Function: Include antioxidant-rich foods (such as berries and leafy greens) and omega-3 fatty acids to support brain health and cognitive function.

CONCLUSION
Midlife nutrition plays a pivotal role in maintaining health, managing weight, and reducing the risk of age-related health conditions. By focusing on a balanced diet rich in essential nutrients, staying physically active, managing stress, and seeking regular healthcare screenings, individuals can optimize their health and well-being during this transformative stage of life. Remember, making informed nutritional choices now can contribute to a vibrant and healthy future.

MENOPAUSE AND BEYOND: ADAPTING TO CHANGING NUTRITIONAL NEEDS
Menopause marks a significant transition in a woman's life, typically occurring around the age of 50. This stage brings about hormonal changes that can affect metabolism, bone health, and overall well-being. Proper nutrition during and after menopause plays a crucial role in managing symptoms, supporting bone health, and promoting overall vitality. This chapter explores the nutritional needs of women during and beyond menopause, strategies for adapting to hormonal changes, and practical tips for maintaining optimal health.

NUTRITIONAL NEEDS DURING MENOPAUSE
During menopause, estrogen levels decline, leading to changes in metabolism and nutrient requirements. Key nutritional considerations include:

1. Calcium and Vitamin D: Essential for maintaining bone health and reducing the risk of osteoporosis.

Recommendation: Aim for 1,200 mg of calcium per day and 600-800 IU of vitamin D.

2. Protein: Important for preserving muscle mass, which can decline with age and hormonal changes.

Recommendation: Include lean sources such as poultry, fish, beans, and tofu.

3. Omega-3 Fatty Acids: Support heart health and may help alleviate symptoms like hot flashes.

Sources: Fatty fish (like salmon), flaxseeds, chia seeds, and walnuts.

4. Fiber: Crucial for digestive health, managing cholesterol levels, and promoting satiety.

Recommendation: Aim for at least 25 grams of fiber per day from fruits, vegetables, whole grains, and legumes.

5. Phytoestrogens: Found in foods like soybeans, flaxseeds, and whole grains, these compounds may help alleviate menopausal symptoms by mimicking estrogen in the body.

ADAPTING TO HORMONAL CHANGES
During and after menopause, women may experience various symptoms and changes that can impact their nutritional needs:

1. Weight Management: Hormonal changes can lead to weight gain, particularly around the abdomen. Focus on portion control and choosing nutrient-dense foods to manage weight.

2. Bone Health: Declining estrogen levels increase the risk of osteoporosis. Incorporate calcium-rich foods and weight-bearing exercises to support bone density.

3. Heart Health: Menopause is associated with an increased risk of cardiovascular disease. Prioritize heart-healthy fats, limit saturated and trans fats, and monitor blood pressure and cholesterol levels.

4. Mental Health: Hormonal fluctuations may affect mood and cognitive function. Include foods rich in omega-3 fatty acids and antioxidants to support brain health.

PRACTICAL TIPS FOR MAINTAINING HEALTH
1. Balanced Diet: Emphasize whole foods, including fruits, vegetables, whole grains, lean proteins, and healthy fats.
Meal Planning: Plan meals ahead to ensure balanced nutrition and avoid processed foods.

2. Hydration: Drink plenty of water to support overall health and alleviate symptoms like dryness.

3. Physical Activity: Include regular aerobic exercise, strength training, and flexibility exercises to support metabolism, bone health, and overall well-being.

4. Stress Management: Practice stress-reducing techniques such as yoga, meditation, or deep breathing exercises to support hormonal balance and mental well-being.

5. Regular Health Screenings: Schedule regular check-ups with healthcare providers to monitor bone density, cholesterol levels, and other health markers.

ADDRESSING COMMON CONCERNS

1. Hot Flashes: Some women find relief by avoiding triggers like caffeine, spicy foods, and alcohol. Maintaining a healthy weight and staying hydrated may also help.

2. Sleep Disturbances: Incorporate relaxation techniques, maintain a consistent sleep schedule, and avoid large meals and caffeine before bedtime.

3. Bone Density: Discuss calcium and vitamin D supplementation with your healthcare provider if dietary intake is inadequate.

CONCLUSION
Navigating menopause and the years beyond requires adapting to changing nutritional needs and focusing on overall health and well-being. By prioritizing a balanced diet, regular physical activity, stress management, and seeking regular healthcare guidance, women can effectively manage symptoms, support bone health, and promote vitality during this transformative stage of life. Remember, each woman's experience with menopause is unique, so personalized nutritional strategies and lifestyle adjustments can help optimize health and quality of life.

SPECIAL CONSIDERATIONS

PLANT-BASED DIETS: VEGETARIAN AND VEGAN NUTRITION

Plant-based diets, including vegetarian and vegan lifestyles, have gained popularity for their health benefits, environmental sustainability, and ethical considerations. This chapter explores the nutritional principles of plant-based diets, the benefits and challenges of vegetarian and vegan nutrition, and practical tips for achieving balanced and nutrient-rich meals.

UNDERSTANDING PLANT-BASED DIETS
Plant-based diets focus primarily on foods derived from plants, including fruits, vegetables, grains, legumes, nuts, seeds, and oils. There are several variations:

1. Vegetarian Diet:

Lacto-ovo-vegetarian: Includes dairy and eggs but excludes meat, poultry, and seafood.
Lacto-vegetarian: Includes dairy but excludes eggs, meat, poultry, and seafood.
Ovo-vegetarian: Includes eggs but excludes dairy, meat, poultry, and seafood.
Pescatarian: Includes seafood but excludes meat and poultry.

2. Vegan Diet:

Excludes all animal products, including meat, poultry, seafood, dairy, eggs, and sometimes honey.

NUTRITIONAL CONSIDERATIONS
Plant-based diets offer numerous health benefits when well-planned, but require attention to certain nutrients:

1. Protein:

Sources: Legumes (beans, lentils), soy products (tofu, tempeh), nuts, seeds, and whole grains.
Combining: Consuming a variety of protein sources throughout the day ensures adequate intake of essential amino acids.

2. Iron:

Sources: Legumes, tofu, nuts, seeds, whole grains, and fortified cereals.
Enhancing Absorption: Pair iron-rich foods with vitamin C sources (citrus fruits, tomatoes) to enhance absorption.

3. Calcium:

Sources: Fortified plant-based milk (soy, almond), tofu (made with calcium sulfate), leafy greens (kale, collard greens).
Absorption: Ensure adequate vitamin D intake to support calcium absorption.

4. Vitamin B12:

Sources: Fortified foods (plant-based milk, nutritional yeast) or supplements for vegans. Lacto-ovo vegetarians can get B12 from dairy and eggs.

5. Omega-3 Fatty Acids:

Sources: Flaxseeds, chia seeds, walnuts, and algae-derived supplements for vegans.

6. Vitamin D:

Sources: Sunlight exposure, fortified plant-based milk, and supplements as needed.

BENEFITS OF PLANT-BASED DIETs

1. Health Benefits: Lower risk of chronic diseases such as heart disease, hypertension, type 2 diabetes, and certain cancers.

2. Weight Management: Plant-based diets tend to be lower in calories and saturated fats, promoting weight loss and maintenance.

3. Environmental Sustainability: Reduced environmental impact through lower greenhouse gas emissions and water usage compared to animal-based diets.

4. Ethical Considerations: Aligns with animal welfare concerns and ethical beliefs regarding animal exploitation.

CHALLENGES AND PRACTICAL TIPS

1. Nutrient Planning: Careful meal planning to ensure adequate intake of protein, iron, calcium, vitamin B12, and omega-3 fatty acids.

2. Variety: Embrace a wide variety of plant foods to maximize nutrient diversity and enjoyment.

3. Fortification and Supplements: Consider fortified foods and supplements to meet specific nutrient needs, especially vitamin B12 and vitamin D.

4. Cooking Methods: Explore different cooking techniques (roasting, steaming, sautéing) to enhance flavors and textures of plant-based meals.

5. Dining Out: Research restaurant menus for plant-based options or modifications, and communicate dietary preferences to servers.

CONCLUSION
Plant-based diets, whether vegetarian or vegan, offer a wealth of health benefits when well-planned and balanced. By focusing on nutrient-dense foods, incorporating a variety of plant sources, and addressing specific nutrient needs through fortification and supplementation as necessary, individuals can thrive on a plant-based lifestyle. Whether motivated by health, environmental concerns, or ethical beliefs, embracing plant-based nutrition can contribute to a sustainable and fulfilling dietary approach.

MANAGING FOOD ALLERGIES AND INTOLERANCES
Food allergies and intolerances affect millions of people worldwide, influencing dietary choices and impacting overall health and well-being. This chapter explores the differences between food allergies and intolerances, common allergens and intolerant foods, strategies for managing these conditions, and practical tips for navigating daily life with dietary restrictions.

UNDERSTANDING FOOD ALLERGIES AND INTOLERANCES

1. Food Allergies:

Definition: Food allergies involve the immune system reacting to specific proteins in food, triggering symptoms that can range from mild to severe (anaphylaxis).
Common Allergens: Peanuts, tree nuts, milk, eggs, wheat, soy, fish, and shellfish.
Symptoms: Itchy skin, hives, swelling, difficulty breathing, and digestive issues.
Management: Strict avoidance of allergenic foods, carrying emergency medications (e.g., epinephrine auto-injector), and seeking medical advice for diagnosis and management.

2. Food Intolerances:

Definition: Food intolerances involve difficulty digesting certain foods, leading to symptoms like bloating, gas, diarrhea, or headaches.
Common Intolerances: Lactose (dairy), gluten (wheat, barley, rye), histamine (aged cheeses, fermented foods), and FODMAPs (certain carbohydrates like onions, garlic).
Symptoms: Digestive discomfort, headaches, skin reactions, and fatigue.
Management: Limiting or avoiding trigger foods, identifying personal tolerance levels, and working with healthcare providers or dietitians for guidance.

STRATEGIES FOR MANAGING FOOD ALLERGIES AND INTOLERANCES

1. Read Labels Carefully:

Allergens: Look for allergen labeling on packaged foods and avoid cross-contamination risks.
Ingredients: Understand food labels for hidden sources of allergens or intolerant substances.

2. Plan Meals and Snacks:

Home Cooking: Prepare meals from scratch to control ingredients and avoid allergens or intolerant foods.
Batch Cooking: Cook in bulk and freeze portions to have safe meals readily available.

3. Communication:

Restaurants: Inform servers about allergies or intolerances when dining out, ask about ingredient details, and request modifications if needed.
Social Gatherings: Communicate dietary restrictions to hosts or bring safe foods to events.

4. Alternative Ingredients:

Substitutions: Use allergy-friendly or tolerated alternatives in recipes, such as dairy-free milk, gluten-free grains, or egg replacers.

5. Education and Support:

Healthcare Professionals: Consult allergists, dietitians, or nutritionists for personalized advice and management plans.
Support Groups: Join online or local support groups for individuals with similar dietary restrictions for shared experiences and tips.

PRACTICAL TIPS FOR DAILY LIVING

1. Traveling: Research safe dining options, pack allergen-free snacks, and carry medications or allergy cards in multiple languages if traveling abroad.

2. School or Workplace:

Education: Educate teachers, coworkers, or supervisors about allergies or intolerances.
Emergency Plans: Develop action plans for emergencies and ensure access to medications (e.g., epinephrine) if necessary.

3. Cross-Contamination Awareness:
Kitchen Safety: Use separate utensils, cutting boards, and cooking surfaces for allergen-free meal preparation.

Labeling: Clearly mark allergen-free foods in shared spaces like refrigerators or pantries.

EMOTIONAL AND SOCIAL CONSIDERATIONS

1. Psychological Impact: Manage stress related to dietary restrictions through mindfulness, support networks, and counseling if needed.

2. Social Interactions:

Inclusivity: Advocate for understanding among friends, family, and colleagues to accommodate dietary needs.
Celebrations: Plan ahead for safe options during holidays and celebrations.

CONCLUSION
Managing food allergies and intolerances requires diligence, education, and proactive planning to maintain health and quality of life. By understanding the differences between allergies and intolerances, implementing strategies for safe eating, and seeking support from healthcare professionals and communities, individuals can navigate daily challenges and enjoy a fulfilling, allergen-conscious lifestyle. Remember, effective management involves collaboration with healthcare providers, informed decision-making, and fostering supportive environments in both personal and social settings.

NUTRITION FOR ATHLETIC PERFORMANCE
Nutrition plays a fundamental role in optimizing athletic performance, supporting recovery, and enhancing overall health and well-being. This chapter explores the key principles of nutrition for athletes, strategies for fueling workouts, recovery nutrition, hydration, and practical tips for achieving peak performance.

KEY PRINCIPLES OF SPORTS NUTRITION

1. Macronutrients:

Carbohydrates: Provide energy for exercise, particularly during high-intensity and endurance activities.
Sources: Whole grains, fruits, vegetables, and legumes.

Proteins: Essential for muscle repair, growth, and maintenance.
Sources: Lean meats, poultry, fish, dairy, eggs, legumes, and plant-based proteins (tofu, tempeh).

Fats: Provide sustained energy and support overall health.
Sources: Healthy fats from avocados, nuts, seeds, olive oil, and fatty fish (like salmon).

2. Micronutrients:

Vitamins and Minerals: Support various physiological functions and play roles in energy metabolism, muscle function, and immune health.
Sources: Fruits, vegetables, whole grains, nuts, seeds, and lean proteins.

3. Hydration:

Importance: Maintain fluid balance, regulate body temperature, and support nutrient transport and digestion.
Guidelines: Drink fluids before, during, and after exercise to prevent dehydration. Water is generally sufficient for hydration, but electrolyte-rich beverages may be beneficial during prolonged or intense workouts.

4. Timing and Composition of Meals:

Pre-Exercise: Consume a balanced meal or snack containing carbohydrates and a moderate amount of protein 2-3 hours before exercise to fuel muscles and optimize performance.
During Exercise: For endurance activities lasting longer than 60-90 minutes, consider consuming easily digestible carbohydrates (e.g., sports drinks, energy gels) to maintain blood glucose levels and sustain performance.
Post-Exercise: Replenish glycogen stores and support muscle repair by consuming a meal or snack containing carbohydrates and protein within 30-60 minutes after exercise.
Strategies for Fueling Workouts

1. Carbohydrate Loading:
Endurance Events: For events lasting longer than 90 minutes, athletes may benefit from carbohydrate loading in the days leading up to the event to maximize glycogen stores.

2. Protein Needs:
Muscle Repair: Consume protein-rich foods throughout the day, especially post-exercise, to support muscle recovery and growth.

3. Healthy Fats:
Sustained Energy: Include sources of healthy fats in meals to provide long-lasting energy and support overall health.

RECOVERY NUTRITION
1. Carbohydrates:
Restore Glycogen: Consume carbohydrates post-exercise to replenish glycogen stores and promote recovery.

2. Protein:
Muscle Repair: Include protein-rich foods or supplements to support muscle repair and growth.

3. Fluids and Electrolytes:
Rehydrate: Drink fluids and electrolyte-rich beverages to replace losses from sweat and maintain hydration status.

PRACTICAL TIPS FOR ATHLETES

1. Individualized Nutrition Plans:
Consultation: Work with a sports dietitian or nutritionist to develop personalized nutrition plans based on training goals, sport-specific demands, and individual preferences.

2. Balanced Diet:
Variety: Incorporate a variety of nutrient-dense foods to ensure adequate intake of vitamins, minerals, and antioxidants.

3. Supplements:
Caution: Use supplements judiciously and under the guidance of a healthcare professional or sports dietitian to address specific nutrient needs that cannot be met through diet alone.

4. Monitoring Performance and Recovery:
Feedback: Pay attention to how different foods and hydration strategies impact performance and recovery. Adjust nutrition plans accordingly.

CONCLUSION

Nutrition is a cornerstone of athletic performance, influencing energy levels, recovery, and overall health. By understanding the principles of sports nutrition, including macronutrient needs, hydration strategies, and the importance of timing and composition of meals, athletes can optimize their performance and achieve their goals. With personalized nutrition plans, attention to hydration, and thoughtful meal planning, athletes can support their bodies' demands and enhance their competitive edge in sports and fitness activities.

UNDERSTANDING AND MANAGING WEIGHT

Weight management is a complex interplay of nutrition, physical activity, metabolism, and lifestyle factors. This chapter explores the principles of weight management, strategies for achieving and maintaining a healthy weight, factors influencing weight gain and loss, and practical tips for sustainable behavior change.

PRINCIPLES OF WEIGHT MANAGEMENT

1. Energy Balance:
Calories In vs. Calories Out: Achieving a healthy weight involves balancing the energy (calories) consumed through food and beverages with the energy expended through metabolism and physical activity.

2. Macronutrients:

Balanced Diet: Emphasize whole foods, including fruits, vegetables, lean proteins, whole grains, and healthy fats, to support overall health and satiety.
Portion Control: Pay attention to portion sizes to avoid overconsumption of calories.

3. Physical Activity:

Exercise: Incorporate regular aerobic exercise, strength training, and flexibility exercises to support calorie expenditure, muscle maintenance, and overall health.

4. Behavior Change:

Lifestyle Habits: Adopt sustainable habits such as mindful eating, regular meal patterns, adequate sleep, stress management, and hydration.

FACTORS INFLUENCING WEIGHT

1. Metabolism:

Basal Metabolic Rate (BMR): The energy expended at rest to maintain basic physiological functions.
Factors: Age, sex, genetics, muscle mass, and hormonal factors influence metabolism.

2. Hormones:

Leptin and Ghrelin: Hormones that regulate hunger and appetite, influencing food intake and energy balance.
Insulin: Regulates blood sugar levels and fat storage.

3. Genetics and Environment:

Genetic Predisposition: Family history may influence weight tendencies.
Environment: Access to healthy foods, socioeconomic factors, cultural influences, and social support impact dietary choices and physical activity levels.

STRATEGIES FOR ACHIEVING AND MAINTAINING A HEALTHY WEIGHT
1. Set Realistic Goals:
SMART Goals: Specific, Measurable, Achievable, Relevant, and Time-bound goals for weight loss or maintenance.

2. Nutrition:
Caloric Deficit: To lose weight, create a modest caloric deficit through a balanced diet and portion control.
Healthy Eating: Focus on nutrient-dense foods and limit added sugars, refined grains, and unhealthy fats.

3. Physical Activity:
Exercise Routine: Combine aerobic exercise (e.g., walking, jogging, swimming) with strength training (e.g., weight lifting, resistance exercises) for optimal weight management and overall health.

4. Behavior Modification:
Mindful Eating: Pay attention to hunger and fullness cues, avoid emotional eating, and practice portion control.
Meal Planning: Plan meals and snacks in advance to support healthy choices and avoid impulsive eating.

5. Support and Accountability:
Social Support: Engage with friends, family, or support groups to stay motivated and accountable.
Professional Guidance: Consult with healthcare providers, registered dietitians, or nutritionists for personalized advice and support.

PRACTICAL TIPS FOR SUSTAINABLE WEIGHT MANAGEMENT
1. Monitor Progress:

Track Food Intake: Use a food diary or mobile app to monitor calorie intake and nutrient consumption.
Track Physical Activity: Keep a log of exercise sessions and physical activity levels.

2. Focus on Long-Term Habits:

Lifestyle Changes: Adopt sustainable habits that promote health and well-being beyond weight loss goals.
Behavioral Strategies: Identify triggers for unhealthy eating habits and develop strategies to overcome challenges.
3. Celebrate Successes:

Non-Scale Victories: Acknowledge achievements such as improved energy levels, mood, and fitness milestones.

CONCLUSION
Understanding and managing weight involves a multifaceted approach that integrates nutrition, physical activity, behavior change, and environmental factors. By embracing principles of energy

balance, adopting healthy eating habits, incorporating regular physical activity, and cultivating supportive behaviors, individuals can achieve and maintain a healthy weight sustainably. With personalized strategies and a commitment to long-term health, successful weight management can enhance overall well-being and quality of life.

NUTRITION FOR MENTAL HEALTH: FOOD AND MOOD
Nutrition plays a crucial role in mental health, influencing mood, cognition, and overall well-being. This chapter explores the connection between diet and mental health, the impact of nutrients on brain function, dietary strategies to support emotional well-being, and practical tips for incorporating mood-boosting foods into daily life.

THE CONNECTION BETWEEN DIET AND MENTAL HEALTH

1. Gut-Brain Axis:

Microbiota: The gut microbiota influence brain function and mood through the production of neurotransmitters like serotonin and dopamine.
Impact of Diet: A balanced diet rich in fiber and probiotics supports a healthy gut microbiome, contributing to improved mental health.

2. Neurotransmitters:

Serotonin: Regulates mood, sleep, and appetite. Precursors include tryptophan-rich foods (e.g., turkey, nuts, seeds).
Dopamine: Influences motivation, reward, and pleasure. Sources include tyrosine-rich foods (e.g., eggs, dairy, tofu).

3. Inflammation and Oxidative Stress:

Antioxidants: Found in colorful fruits and vegetables, antioxidants combat oxidative stress and inflammation linked to mental health disorders.
Omega-3 Fatty Acids: Reduce inflammation and support brain health. Sources include fatty fish (e.g., salmon, sardines), flaxseeds, and walnuts.

NUTRIENTS AND THEIR IMPACT ON MENTAL HEALTH
1. Complex Carbohydrates:

Stabilize Blood Sugar: Whole grains, fruits, and vegetables provide sustained energy and support a stable mood.

2. Protein:
Amino Acids: Precursors to neurotransmitters like serotonin and dopamine. Include lean meats, poultry, fish, beans, and legumes.

3. Healthy Fats:

Omega-3 Fatty Acids: Support brain structure and function, reducing symptoms of depression and anxiety.
Sources: Fatty fish (e.g., salmon, mackerel), flaxseeds, chia seeds, and walnuts.

4. Vitamins and Minerals:

B Vitamins: Support neurotransmitter synthesis and energy production. Sources include whole grains, leafy greens, and fortified foods.
Vitamin D: Linked to mood regulation. Obtain from sunlight exposure and fortified foods (e.g., fortified dairy or plant-based milks, fatty fish).
Magnesium: Supports relaxation and stress management. Found in nuts, seeds, legumes, and leafy greens.

Dietary Strategies for Emotional Well-Being
1. Mediterranean Diet:

Emphasis: High intake of fruits, vegetables, whole grains, nuts, seeds, olive oil, and moderate consumption of fish, poultry, and dairy.
Benefits: Associated with reduced risk of depression and improved mental health outcomes.

2. Probiotics and Prebiotics:

Probiotics: Found in fermented foods like yogurt, kefir, kimchi, and sauerkraut, support gut health and mental well-being.
Prebiotics: Found in fiber-rich foods like onions, garlic, bananas, and oats, nourish beneficial gut bacteria.

3. Hydration:
Importance: Dehydration can affect mood and cognitive function. Drink adequate water throughout the day.

PRACTICAL TIPS FOR INCORPORATING MOOD-BOOSTING FOODS

1. Balanced Meals:

Include a variety of nutrient-dense foods: Fruits, vegetables, whole grains, lean proteins, and healthy fats in each meal.

2. Snack Smart:

Healthy Options: Choose snacks rich in nutrients such as nuts, seeds, yogurt, or fresh fruits.

3. Mindful Eating:

Awareness: Pay attention to hunger and fullness cues, and savor the flavors and textures of food.

4. Limit Sugar and Processed Foods:

Impact on Mood: Reduce consumption of sugary snacks and processed foods that can lead to energy crashes and mood swings.

CONCLUSION
Nutrition significantly influences mental health and emotional well-being by supporting neurotransmitter function, reducing inflammation, and promoting a healthy gut-brain connection. By incorporating nutrient-rich foods, adopting dietary patterns like the Mediterranean diet, and prioritizing hydration and gut health, individuals can optimize their mood and cognitive function. Making informed food choices and embracing a balanced approach to eating not only supports mental health but enhances overall quality of life.

PRACTICAL TIPS AND STRATEGIES

MEAL PLANNING AND PREPARATION
Effective meal planning and preparation are essential for maintaining a nutritious diet, saving time and money, and reducing stress around mealtimes. This chapter delves into the benefits of meal planning, steps to create a meal plan, tips for efficient meal preparation, and strategies to make healthy eating convenient and enjoyable.

BENEFITS OF MEAL PLANNING AND PREPARATION

1. Nutritional Balance:

Ensures a variety of nutrients in your diet by including different food groups.
Helps avoid last-minute unhealthy food choices.

2. Time and Money Savings:

Reduces the need for frequent grocery shopping and minimizes food waste.
Allows for bulk buying and cooking, saving money and time.

3. Stress Reduction:

Eases the daily decision-making process about what to eat.
Provides peace of mind knowing that meals are planned and ready.

4. Portion Control:

Helps manage portion sizes, supporting weight management and nutritional goals.

5. Customization:

Allows for the inclusion of personal preferences and dietary requirements, ensuring meals meet individual health needs.

STEPS TO CREATE A MEAL PLAN

1. Assess Your Needs:

Health Goals: Identify specific dietary goals (e.g., weight loss, muscle gain, improved energy).
Dietary Preferences and Restrictions: Consider allergies, intolerances, and personal preferences.

2. Plan for the Week:

Meals and Snacks: Plan all meals and snacks for the week to ensure a balanced diet.
Variety: Include a mix of proteins, carbohydrates, and healthy fats, along with plenty of fruits and vegetables.

3. Create a Shopping List:

Ingredients: List all ingredients needed for the planned meals, organized by category (e.g., produce, dairy, grains).
Staples: Keep a stock of pantry staples (e.g., spices, oils, canned goods) for easy meal preparation.

4. Schedule Preparation Time:

Cooking Sessions: Dedicate specific times during the week for meal prep (e.g., Sunday afternoon).
Batch Cooking: Cook large batches of grains, proteins, and vegetables that can be used in various meals.

TIPS FOR EFFICIENT MEAL PREPARATION

1. Prepare in Batches:

Cook Once, Eat Multiple Times: Prepare large quantities of staple foods like rice, quinoa, chicken, and roasted vegetables.
Freezing: Portion and freeze meals for easy reheating on busy days.

2. Use Time-Saving Appliances:

Slow Cooker/Instant Pot: Utilize these appliances for hands-off cooking.
Blender/Food Processor: Speed up preparation of smoothies, sauces, and chopped vegetables.

3. Pre-Portion Meals:

Containers: Use portion-controlled containers to store meals and snacks, making them easy to grab and go.
Labeling: Label containers with the contents and date to keep track of freshness.

4. Simplify Recipes:

Easy-to-Make: Choose recipes with fewer ingredients and straightforward instructions.

Versatile Ingredients: Select ingredients that can be used in multiple dishes to minimize complexity.

5. Plan for Leftovers:

Repurpose: Transform leftovers into new meals (e.g., roasted vegetables into a stir-fry, grilled chicken into a salad).

STRATEGIES FOR HEALTHY EATING CONVENIENCE

1. Healthy Snack Prep:

Fruits and Vegetables: Pre-wash and cut fruits and vegetables for quick snacks.
Protein Snacks: Prepare protein-rich snacks like boiled eggs, yogurt, and hummus with veggies.

2. Overnight Meals:

Overnight Oats: Combine oats, milk (or plant-based alternative), fruits, and nuts in a jar for a ready-to-eat breakfast.
Marinated Proteins: Marinate proteins overnight for flavorful, ready-to-cook meals.

3. Build a Meal Prep Routine:

Consistency: Establish a regular meal prep routine that fits your schedule.
Adjust as Needed: Be flexible and adjust your meal prep routine based on your lifestyle and needs.

4. Stay Organized:

Kitchen Organization: Keep your kitchen organized and stocked with essentials to streamline meal prep.
Grocery Shopping: Stick to your shopping list to avoid impulse buys and ensure you have all necessary ingredients.

CONCLUSION
Meal planning and preparation are powerful tools for achieving and maintaining a healthy diet. By taking the time to plan meals, create a shopping list, and prepare ingredients in advance, you can enjoy balanced, nutritious meals with less stress and effort. Implementing these strategies can lead to improved health outcomes, better time management, and a more enjoyable eating experience. Embrace meal planning and preparation as part of your routine to support your overall well-being and dietary goals.

READING FOOD LABELS: MAKING INFORMED CHOICES

Understanding food labels is essential for making informed choices that support your health and nutritional goals. This chapter covers the key components of food labels, how to interpret them, and practical tips for using this information to make healthier choices.

KEY COMPONENTS OF FOOD LABELS

1. Nutrition Facts Panel:

Serving Size: Indicates the amount of food that constitutes one serving and helps determine the nutrient content per serving.
Calories: Shows the amount of energy provided per serving.
Macronutrients: Lists the grams of total fat, saturated fat, trans fat, cholesterol, sodium, total carbohydrates, dietary fiber, total sugars, added sugars, and protein.
Micronutrients: Includes vitamins and minerals, such as vitamin D, calcium, iron, and potassium, presented as a percentage of the Daily Value (DV).

2. Ingredient List:

Order of Ingredients: Ingredients are listed in descending order by weight, with the most abundant ingredient first.
Additives and Preservatives: Identifies any artificial or natural additives, preservatives, and flavorings.

3. Allergen Information:

Common Allergens: Highlights the presence of common allergens such as peanuts, tree nuts, soy, wheat, dairy, eggs, fish, and shellfish.

4. Nutrient Claims:

Health Claims: Statements about the health benefits of the product, such as "low fat," "high fiber," or "supports heart health," which are regulated by health authorities.
Nutrient Content Claims: Describes the level of a nutrient in the product, such as "low sodium" or "sugar-free."

HOW TO INTERPRET FOOD LABELS

1. Serving Size and Servings Per Container:

Check Serving Size: Compare the serving size on the label to the amount you actually eat. Many packages contain more than one serving.
Total Servings: Multiply the nutrient values by the number of servings you consume to get the total intake.

2. Calories:

Caloric Needs: Align your calorie intake with your daily caloric needs based on your activity level, age, and health goals.

3. Macronutrients:

Fat: Aim for products low in saturated and trans fats to support heart health.
Carbohydrates: Look for products with whole grains and high dietary fiber content. Be mindful of added sugars.
Protein: Check the protein content, especially if you need more protein for muscle maintenance or growth.

4. Micronutrients:

Daily Values: Use the %DV to gauge how much of a nutrient a serving of the food contributes to your daily intake. Aim for higher %DV for vitamins, minerals, and fiber and lower %DV for saturated fat, cholesterol, and sodium.

5. Ingredients:

First Few Ingredients: The first three ingredients are the most significant. Look for whole, unprocessed ingredients.
Avoid Harmful Additives: Be cautious of ingredients you want to limit, such as high fructose corn syrup, artificial colors, and preservatives.

6. Allergen Information:

Safety: Always check for allergens if you have food allergies or intolerances to avoid adverse reactions.

PRACTICAL TIPS FOR MAKING HEALTHIER CHOICES
1. Compare Labels:

Product Comparison: When choosing between similar products, compare their Nutrition Facts Panels and ingredient lists to find the healthier option.
Nutrient Density: Opt for foods that offer more nutrients (vitamins, minerals, fiber) for fewer calories.

2. Watch for Hidden Sugars:

Multiple Names: Added sugars can be listed under various names, such as sucrose, fructose, corn syrup, and honey. Be mindful of the total amount of added sugars.

3. Understand Marketing Terms:

Buzzwords: Terms like "natural," "multigrain," and "organic" can be misleading. Always read the Nutrition Facts Panel and ingredient list to verify the healthfulness of the product.

4. Portion Control:

Serving Sizes: Use the serving size information to control portions and avoid overeating.

5. Balance and Moderation:

Dietary Balance: Choose a variety of foods to ensure a balanced intake of all necessary nutrients.
Occasional Treats: It's okay to enjoy less healthy foods occasionally, but make sure they are part of an overall balanced diet.

CONCLUSION
Reading food labels is a valuable skill for making informed dietary choices. By understanding the components of food labels and knowing how to interpret them, you can better manage your nutritional intake, support your health goals, and make smarter food choices. Incorporate these practices into your shopping routine to empower yourself with knowledge and improve your overall diet and well-being.

DINING OUT AND TRAVELING: STAYING ON TRACK
Maintaining a healthy diet while dining out and traveling can be challenging, but it is entirely achievable with some planning and mindful choices. This chapter offers strategies for staying on track with your nutritional goals when eating at restaurants or on the go, practical tips for making healthier choices, and advice for preparing in advance to ensure you stay nourished and satisfied.

STRATEGIES FOR DINING OUT

1. Plan Ahead:

Research Menus: Look up restaurant menus online before you go. Identify healthy options or dishes that can be modified to suit your dietary needs.
Meal Timing: Plan your meals around your dining out schedule to avoid overeating. If you know you're dining out for dinner, have a lighter lunch and a healthy snack.

2. Make Healthier Choices:

Vegetables First: Choose dishes that are rich in vegetables, whether it's a salad, stir-fry, or a side of steamed veggies.

Lean Proteins: Opt for grilled, baked, or steamed proteins like chicken, fish, or plant-based alternatives over fried or breaded options.
Whole Grains: Select whole grain options like brown rice, quinoa, or whole wheat bread when available.

3. Portion Control:

Appetizers as Main Course: Consider ordering an appetizer as your main course or splitting an entrée with a friend to control portions.
Side Salads and Soups: Start with a side salad or a broth-based soup to help fill you up and reduce the likelihood of overeating.
Take Home Leftovers: If portions are large, ask for a to-go box at the beginning of the meal and pack half of it away for later.

4. Mindful Eating:

Slow Down: Eat slowly and savor each bite. This gives your body time to signal fullness.
Avoid Distractions: Focus on your meal and company rather than screens or other distractions to enhance the dining experience and prevent overeating.

5. Special Requests:

Customization: Don't be afraid to ask for modifications like dressing on the side, steamed instead of sautéed, or substituting vegetables for fries.
Healthier Preparations: Request for meals to be prepared with less oil, butter, or salt.

TIPS FOR TRAVELING

1. Pack Healthy Snacks:

Non-Perishable Options: Carry snacks like nuts, seeds, dried fruit, whole grain crackers, and protein bars.
Fresh Options: If you have access to a cooler, pack fresh fruits, vegetables, yogurt, and hummus.

2. Stay Hydrated:

Water Bottle: Bring a reusable water bottle and refill it regularly to stay hydrated.
Limit Sugary Drinks: Avoid sugary drinks and opt for water, herbal tea, or seltzer.

3. Smart Choices at Airports and Rest Stops:

Airport Food: Look for healthy options like salads, fresh fruit, yogurt, and lean protein dishes.

Rest Stops: Choose items like fruit cups, pre-packaged salads, and grilled chicken sandwiches from fast-food restaurants.

4. Hotel Strategies:

Healthy Breakfast: Take advantage of hotel breakfasts by choosing oatmeal, fresh fruit, eggs, and whole grain toast.
In-Room Options: Stock your hotel room with healthy snacks and consider using the microwave for simple meals.

5. Eating Out While Traveling:

Local Markets: Explore local markets for fresh produce, local specialties, and healthier options.
Balance: Balance indulgent meals with lighter, healthier ones. If you have a heavy dinner planned, opt for a lighter lunch.

PREPARING IN ADVANCE
1. Research and Plan:

Destination Research: Research food options at your destination to find healthy eateries and markets.
Meal Plan: If possible, plan some meals and snacks ahead of time to reduce reliance on less healthy convenience foods.

2. Pack Essentials:

Travel Utensils: Bring portable utensils, a small cutting board, and containers for easy meal prep.
Supplements: If needed, pack any dietary supplements to ensure you meet your nutritional needs.

3. Stay Active:

Exercise Routine: Incorporate physical activity into your travel plans, whether it's a morning walk, a workout at the hotel gym, or exploring the area by bike.

CONCLUSION
Dining out and traveling don't have to derail your healthy eating habits. By planning ahead, making mindful choices, and preparing for potential challenges, you can stay on track with your nutritional goals while enjoying new experiences and flavors. Embrace these strategies to maintain balance, nourish your body, and enjoy your meals wherever you are.

SUPPLEMENTS: WHEN AND WHAT TO CONSIDER

While a well-balanced diet should be the primary source of nutrients, supplements can play a valuable role in ensuring you meet your nutritional needs, especially when certain conditions or life stages increase nutrient requirements. This chapter discusses when to consider taking supplements, the types of supplements available, guidelines for choosing quality supplements, and potential risks and considerations.

WHEN TO CONSIDER SUPPLEMENTS

1. Nutrient Deficiencies:

Diagnosed Deficiencies: If you have a diagnosed deficiency (e.g., iron, vitamin D, B12), supplements can help restore levels.

Symptoms of Deficiency: Fatigue, weakness, and other health issues can signal nutrient deficiencies, warranting a medical evaluation.

2. Life Stages and Special Conditions:

Pregnancy and Breastfeeding: Increased needs for folic acid, iron, calcium, and DHA.

Infants and Children: Vitamin D and iron supplements may be recommended.

Older Adults: Calcium, vitamin D, B12, and magnesium needs may increase with age.

3. Dietary Restrictions:

Vegetarians and Vegans: Potential needs for B12, iron, zinc, calcium, and omega-3 fatty acids.

Food Allergies/Intolerances: Supplements can help bridge nutritional gaps caused by restricted diets.

4. Health Conditions:

Chronic Illnesses: Conditions like osteoporosis, anemia, and celiac disease may require supplementation.

Medications: Some medications can interfere with nutrient absorption (e.g., antacids and vitamin B12).

Types of Supplements

1. Multivitamins:

Comprehensive Coverage: Provide a broad spectrum of vitamins and minerals to cover general dietary gaps.

2. Single Nutrient Supplements:

Specific Needs: Target individual deficiencies or increased needs (e.g., iron, vitamin D, calcium).

3. Herbal Supplements:

Natural Remedies: Includes echinacea, ginkgo biloba, and turmeric for various health benefits, though efficacy and safety vary.

4. Protein Supplements:

Protein Powders: Whey, soy, pea, and other plant-based proteins to support muscle maintenance and growth.

5. Omega-3 Fatty Acids:

Fish Oil and Algal Oil: For heart health, brain function, and inflammation reduction.

6. Probiotics:

Gut Health: Live bacteria and yeasts that support a healthy digestive system.

GUIDELINES FOR CHOOSING QUALITY SUPPLEMENTS

1. Research and Recommendations:

Consult Healthcare Providers: Always talk to your doctor or a registered dietitian before starting any supplement.
Evidence-Based: Choose supplements with evidence supporting their efficacy for your specific needs.

2. Quality Assurance:

Third-Party Testing: Look for supplements tested by independent organizations (e.g., USP, NSF, ConsumerLab).
Reputable Brands: Choose brands with good reputations and transparent labeling practices.

3. Label Reading:

Ingredients: Check for active ingredients, dosages, and potential allergens.
Additives: Avoid supplements with unnecessary fillers, artificial colors, and preservatives.

4. Dosage and Form:

Appropriate Dosage: Follow recommended dosages and avoid mega-doses unless prescribed.

Preferred Form: Choose forms that are well-absorbed and convenient for you (e.g., liquid, capsule, chewable).

POTENTIAL RISKS AND CONSIDERATIONS

1. Over-Supplementation:

Toxicity: High doses of certain vitamins and minerals can be toxic (e.g., vitamin A, iron).
Balanced Diet: Relying on supplements can lead to neglecting a balanced diet, which provides other essential nutrients and fiber.

2. Interactions:

Medication Interactions: Supplements can interact with medications, affecting their efficacy or causing side effects.
Nutrient Interactions: Some nutrients can interfere with the absorption or function of others (e.g., calcium and iron).

3. Regulation and Safety:

Lack of Regulation: Supplements are not as strictly regulated as pharmaceuticals, so quality and efficacy can vary.
Recalls and Warnings: Stay informed about recalls and safety warnings for specific supplements.

CONCLUSION
Supplements can be a beneficial addition to your diet, particularly when specific nutritional needs arise due to deficiencies, life stages, dietary restrictions, or health conditions. However, they should complement, not replace, a balanced diet. Always consult with healthcare professionals before starting any supplement regimen, choose high-quality products, and be mindful of potential risks and interactions. By taking a thoughtful approach to supplementation, you can effectively support your overall health and well-being.

RECIPES AND MEAL PLANS

BREAKFAST IDEAS: STARTING YOUR DAY RIGHT

Breakfast is often called the most important meal of the day, and for good reason. A nutritious breakfast can provide the energy and nutrients needed to start the day off right. This chapter offers a variety of breakfast ideas that are quick, easy, and packed with essential nutrients to keep you fueled and focused throughout the morning.

THE IMPORTANCE OF A NUTRITIOUS BREAKFAST

1. Energy Boost:

Refueling: After an overnight fast, breakfast replenishes your body's energy stores.
Sustained Energy: A balanced breakfast with complex carbohydrates, protein, and healthy fats provides steady energy.

2. Cognitive Function:

Improved Concentration: Eating breakfast improves focus, memory, and cognitive performance.
Mood Regulation: A nutritious meal can enhance mood and reduce irritability.

3. Metabolic Benefits:

Kickstarting Metabolism: Eating in the morning helps jumpstart your metabolism and supports healthy weight management.
Blood Sugar Control: A balanced breakfast helps regulate blood sugar levels, preventing mid-morning energy crashes.

QUICK AND NUTRITIOUS BREAKFAST IDEAS
1. Smoothie Bowls:

Ingredients: Blend a base of spinach, kale, or other greens with a banana, berries, Greek yogurt, and a splash of almond milk.
Toppings: Add granola, chia seeds, flaxseeds, and fresh fruit for extra nutrients and texture.

2. Overnight Oats:

Basic Recipe: Combine rolled oats with your choice of milk, yogurt, and a sweetener like honey or maple syrup.
Flavor Variations: Add nuts, seeds, fruits, and spices (e.g., cinnamon, vanilla) for variety. Let it sit in the fridge overnight.

3. Avocado Toast:
Whole Grain Bread: Choose whole grain bread for more fiber and nutrients.
Toppings: Top with mashed avocado, a sprinkle of salt, pepper, and optional additions like cherry tomatoes, poached eggs, or smoked salmon.

4. Yogurt Parfaits:

Layering: Layer Greek yogurt with fresh fruits, granola, and a drizzle of honey.
Nutrient Boost: Add chia seeds, flaxseeds, or a handful of nuts for extra protein and omega-3 fatty acids.

5. Egg Muffins:

Prep Ahead: Whisk eggs with chopped vegetables, cheese, and lean meats. Pour into a muffin tin and bake.
Portion Control: These can be made in advance and reheated for a quick, protein-packed breakfast.

6. Chia Pudding:

Simple Mix: Combine chia seeds with almond milk, vanilla extract, and a sweetener. Let it sit overnight to thicken.
Toppings: Top with fresh fruits, nuts, and a sprinkle of coconut flakes.

7. Whole Grain Pancakes or Waffles:

Healthier Batter: Use whole wheat flour or oat flour in your batter. Add mashed bananas or applesauce for natural sweetness.
Toppings: Top with fresh berries, a dollop of Greek yogurt, and a drizzle of pure maple syrup.

8. Breakfast Burritos:

Filling: Scramble eggs with black beans, bell peppers, onions, and cheese. Wrap in a whole grain tortilla.
Make-Ahead: Freeze individual burritos for a quick, reheatable breakfast option.

9. Fresh Fruit and Nut Butter:

Simple Pairing: Slice an apple or banana and serve with a side of almond butter or peanut butter for a quick and satisfying breakfast.
Additional Toppings: Sprinkle with chia seeds, hemp seeds, or a dash of cinnamon for extra nutrients.

10. Cottage Cheese and Fruit:

Protein-Rich: Pair cottage cheese with fresh fruit like pineapple, berries, or peaches.
Nutrient Boost: Add a handful of nuts or seeds for added crunch and healthy fats.

PRACTICAL TIPS FOR A SUCCESSFUL BREAKFAST ROUTINE

1. Plan Ahead:

Meal Prep: Prepare ingredients or make breakfast items the night before to save time in the morning.
Weekly Planning: Plan a week's worth of breakfasts to ensure variety and balanced nutrition.

2. Balance Your Plate:

Macronutrients: Include a mix of complex carbohydrates, lean protein, and healthy fats in your breakfast.
Fiber-Rich Foods: Incorporate fruits, vegetables, and whole grains to ensure adequate fiber intake.

3. Portion Control:

Moderation: Be mindful of portion sizes to avoid overeating, even with healthy foods.
Listen to Your Body: Eat until you are satisfied, not overly full.

4. Stay Hydrated:

Morning Hydration: Start your day with a glass of water or herbal tea to stay hydrated and support digestion.

5. Adjust to Your Needs:

Customize: Tailor your breakfast choices to your specific dietary needs, preferences, and schedule.
Flexible Timing: If you're not hungry first thing in the morning, have a small snack and a more substantial breakfast later.

CONCLUSION
A nutritious breakfast sets the tone for a productive and energetic day. By incorporating a variety of healthy and delicious breakfast options, you can enjoy the benefits of sustained energy, improved cognitive function, and better overall health. Use these ideas and tips to make breakfast a vital part of your daily routine, ensuring you start each day nourished and ready to take on whatever comes your way.

LUNCH SOLUTIONS: NUTRIENT-PACKED MIDDAY MEALS
Lunch is an essential meal that helps sustain your energy and concentration levels throughout the day. Choosing nutrient-packed options for your midday meal can prevent the afternoon slump and keep you feeling satisfied until dinner. This chapter explores a variety of lunch solutions that are balanced, convenient, and delicious, ensuring you get the nutrients you need to power through your day.

THE IMPORTANCE OF A BALANCED LUNCH

1. Sustained Energy:

Energy Levels: A balanced lunch replenishes energy stores depleted during the morning, helping maintain productivity and focus.
Blood Sugar Stability: Eating a nutrient-dense lunch helps regulate blood sugar levels, preventing energy crashes.

2. Nutritional Balance:

Nutrient Intake: Lunch provides an opportunity to include a variety of food groups, ensuring you meet your daily nutritional requirements.
Healthy Choices: Making conscious choices at lunch can contribute to better overall diet quality and health outcomes.

QUICK AND NUTRITIOUS LUNCH IDEAS

1. Salads:

Base Greens: Use a variety of leafy greens like spinach, kale, arugula, or mixed greens.
Protein Addition: Include lean proteins such as grilled chicken, tofu, beans, or boiled eggs.
Healthy Fats: Add avocado, nuts, seeds, or a drizzle of olive oil.
Whole Grains: Incorporate quinoa, farro, or brown rice for added fiber and nutrients.
Vibrant Veggies: Top with colorful vegetables like bell peppers, cherry tomatoes, cucumbers, and shredded carrots.
Flavor Enhancers: Use herbs, spices, and a homemade vinaigrette for added flavor.

2. Grain Bowls:

Grain Base: Start with a base of brown rice, quinoa, bulgur, or barley.
Protein Source: Add grilled salmon, chickpeas, lentils, or roasted chicken.
Vegetable Variety: Include roasted or steamed vegetables such as broccoli, sweet potatoes, and zucchini.
Tasty Toppings: Sprinkle with feta cheese, nuts, seeds, or a dollop of hummus.

3. Wraps and Sandwiches:

Whole Grain Wraps: Use whole grain tortillas or wraps for added fiber.
Lean Proteins: Fill with turkey, chicken, hummus, or beans.
Fresh Veggies: Add plenty of vegetables like lettuce, tomatoes, cucumbers, and bell peppers.
Healthy Spreads: Use avocado, Greek yogurt-based sauces, or mustard instead of high-fat mayo.

4. Soups and Stews:

Hearty Soups: Prepare soups with a base of broth or tomatoes and include a variety of vegetables, beans, and lean proteins.
Whole Grain Additions: Add whole grains like barley, quinoa, or brown rice to make the soup more filling.
Batch Cooking: Make a large batch and store portions in the freezer for convenient, ready-to-eat meals.

5. Bento Boxes:

Balanced Portions: Include sections for lean protein, whole grains, fresh vegetables, and a small portion of fruit or nuts.
Creative Combinations: Mix and match different ingredients to keep lunches interesting and varied.

6. Stir-Fries:

Quick Cooking: Stir-fry lean proteins like chicken, tofu, or shrimp with a variety of colorful vegetables.
Flavorful Sauces: Use low-sodium soy sauce, garlic, ginger, and a touch of sesame oil for flavor.
Serve with Grains: Pair with brown rice, quinoa, or soba noodles.

7. Leftovers:

Plan Ahead: Cook extra portions at dinner to have leftovers for lunch the next day.
Reinvent Dishes: Repurpose leftovers into new dishes, like turning roasted vegetables and grains into a salad or wrap.

TIPS FOR A SUCCESSFUL LUNCH ROUTINE

1. Meal Prep:

Weekly Preparation: Dedicate a few hours each week to prepare lunch ingredients or complete meals.

Portion Control: Divide meals into individual containers for easy grab-and-go options.

2. Balance Your Plate:

Macronutrients: Ensure each lunch includes a balance of complex carbohydrates, lean proteins, and healthy fats.
Fiber-Rich Foods: Incorporate fiber-rich foods like whole grains, legumes, fruits, and vegetables to aid digestion and keep you full.

3. Mindful Eating:

Take Your Time: Sit down and savor your lunch without distractions to enhance digestion and enjoyment.
Listen to Your Body: Eat until you are satisfied, not overly full.

4. Hydration:

Drink Water: Pair your lunch with a glass of water, herbal tea, or a low-sugar beverage to stay hydrated.

5. Healthy Snacking:

Midday Snacks: If you find yourself hungry between meals, opt for healthy snacks like nuts, fruits, yogurt, or veggie sticks.

6. Variety and Creativity:

Mix It Up: Rotate different recipes and ingredients to keep lunches interesting and prevent monotony.
Explore Cuisines: Try dishes from various cuisines to introduce new flavors and nutrient profiles.

CONCLUSION
A nutrient-packed lunch is crucial for maintaining energy, focus, and overall well-being throughout the day. By incorporating a variety of balanced and delicious lunch options, you can ensure you meet your nutritional needs while enjoying your meals. Use these ideas and tips to create a lunch routine that supports your health, keeps you satisfied, and enhances your daily performance.

DINNER RECIPES: BALANCED AND DELICIOUS EVENING MEALS
Dinner is an opportunity to unwind and enjoy a nutritious meal that replenishes your body after a long day. A well-balanced dinner can support digestion, promote restful sleep, and ensure you meet your nutritional needs. This chapter provides a range of dinner recipes that are both delicious and nutritionally balanced, helping you end your day on a healthy note.

THE IMPORTANCE OF A BALANCED DINNER

1. Nutrient Replenishment:

End-of-Day Nutrition: Dinner helps replenish nutrients depleted throughout the day, providing essential vitamins, minerals, and macronutrients.
Balanced Diet: Ensuring your dinner is balanced with proteins, carbohydrates, and fats supports overall dietary balance.

2. Digestion and Sleep:

Proper Digestion: Eating a nutritious, well-portioned dinner supports healthy digestion.
Restful Sleep: Avoiding heavy, greasy foods and opting for balanced meals can promote better sleep quality.

3. Family and Social Connection:

Quality Time: Dinner is often a time for family and friends to connect, enhancing emotional well-being.

BALANCED AND DELICIOUS DINNER RECIPES

1. Baked Salmon with Quinoa and Steamed Vegetables:

Ingredients:
2 salmon fillets
1 cup quinoa
2 cups mixed vegetables (broccoli, carrots, bell peppers)
Olive oil, lemon juice, garlic, salt, and pepper

Instructions:
Preheat the oven to 400°F (200°C).
Place salmon on a baking sheet, drizzle with olive oil, and season with garlic, lemon juice, salt, and pepper. Bake for 15-20 minutes.
Cook quinoa according to package instructions.
Steam mixed vegetables until tender.
Serve salmon over quinoa with a side of steamed vegetables.

2. Chicken and Vegetable Stir-Fry:

Ingredients:
2 boneless, skinless chicken breasts, sliced
1 cup broccoli florets
1 red bell pepper, sliced

1 carrot, julienned
1 onion, sliced
2 tbsp soy sauce
1 tbsp olive oil
1 tsp ginger, minced
1 garlic clove, minced

Instructions:
Heat olive oil in a large skillet over medium-high heat.
Add chicken slices and cook until no longer pink.
Add garlic, ginger, and vegetables. Stir-fry until vegetables are tender-crisp.
Stir in soy sauce and cook for another 2-3 minutes.
Serve over brown rice or whole grain noodles.

3. Vegetarian Stuffed Peppers:

Ingredients:
4 large bell peppers, tops cut off and seeds removed
1 cup cooked brown rice
1 can black beans, drained and rinsed
1 cup corn kernels
1 cup diced tomatoes
1 tsp cumin
1 tsp chili powder
Salt and pepper to taste
1 cup shredded cheese (optional)

Instructions:
Preheat the oven to 375°F (190°C).
In a large bowl, mix brown rice, black beans, corn, tomatoes, cumin, chili powder, salt, and pepper.
Stuff each bell pepper with the rice mixture and place in a baking dish.
If using, sprinkle cheese on top of each pepper.
Cover with foil and bake for 30 minutes. Remove foil and bake for an additional 10 minutes.
Serve hot with a side salad.

4. Lentil and Sweet Potato Curry:

Ingredients:
1 cup lentils, rinsed
2 sweet potatoes, peeled and diced
1 onion, chopped
2 garlic cloves, minced
1 tbsp curry powder

1 can coconut milk
2 cups vegetable broth
2 cups spinach leaves
Salt and pepper to taste

Instructions:
In a large pot, sauté onion and garlic until fragrant.
Add curry powder and cook for another minute.
Stir in lentils, sweet potatoes, coconut milk, and vegetable broth.
Bring to a boil, then reduce heat and simmer for 20-25 minutes until lentils and sweet potatoes are tender.
Stir in spinach and cook until wilted.
Season with salt and pepper and serve over brown rice or with whole grain naan.

5. Turkey and Avocado Taco Bowls:

Ingredients:
1 lb ground turkey
1 packet taco seasoning
1 cup quinoa, cooked
1 can black beans, drained and rinsed
1 cup corn kernels
1 avocado, diced
1 cup cherry tomatoes, halved
1 cup shredded lettuce
1 lime, cut into wedges
Salsa and Greek yogurt for topping

Instructions:
Cook ground turkey in a skillet until no longer pink. Add taco seasoning and water according to package instructions.
In a bowl, layer quinoa, black beans, corn, turkey, avocado, cherry tomatoes, and shredded lettuce.
Top with salsa and a dollop of Greek yogurt.
Serve with lime wedges on the side.

TIPS FOR A HEALTHY DINNER ROUTINE

1. Plan Ahead:

Weekly Menus: Plan your dinner menu for the week to streamline grocery shopping and meal prep.
Prep Ingredients: Chop vegetables, marinate proteins, and prepare grains ahead of time to save on cooking time.

2. Balance Your Plate:

Macronutrients: Ensure each dinner includes a balance of lean proteins, whole grains, and plenty of vegetables.
Portion Control: Be mindful of portion sizes to avoid overeating, especially late at night.

3. Mindful Eating:

Enjoy Your Meal: Take time to enjoy your dinner, savoring each bite without distractions like TV or smartphones.
Family Meals: Use dinner as an opportunity to connect with family or friends, enhancing both your meal and your social well-being.

4. Hydration:

Drink Water: Pair your dinner with a glass of water or herbal tea to stay hydrated.
Limit Sugary Drinks: Avoid sugary drinks and excessive alcohol consumption during dinner.

5. Post-Dinner Routine:

Light Activity: Engage in light activity, like a walk, after dinner to aid digestion.
Healthy Desserts: If you crave something sweet, opt for healthy dessert options like fruit, yogurt, or a small piece of dark chocolate.

CONCLUSION
A balanced and delicious dinner is key to ending your day on a healthy note. By incorporating a variety of nutritious recipes and maintaining a mindful eating routine, you can ensure that your evening meals support your overall health and well-being. Use these recipes and tips to create satisfying dinners that nourish your body and bring joy to your daily dining experience.

SNACKS AND SMOOTHIES: HEALTHY OPTIONS BETWEEN MEALS
Snacks and smoothies are essential for maintaining energy levels and preventing hunger between meals. Choosing healthy options can keep you satisfied, provide essential nutrients, and support overall well-being. This chapter explores a variety of nutritious snack and smoothie ideas that are easy to prepare and delicious.

THE IMPORTANCE OF HEALTHY SNACKS AND SMOOTHIES

1. Sustained Energy:

Energy Boost: Healthy snacks and smoothies provide a quick energy boost to keep you active and focused throughout the day.

Preventing Crashes: They help maintain stable blood sugar levels, preventing energy crashes and mood swings.

2. Nutrient Intake:

Nutrient-Rich: Snacks and smoothies can be packed with vitamins, minerals, fiber, and protein, contributing to your daily nutrient intake.
Variety: They offer an opportunity to include a wide range of nutrients, especially those you might miss in main meals.

3. Hunger Management:

Appetite Control: Healthy snacks and smoothies help manage hunger, preventing overeating during main meals.
Metabolism Support: Regular, balanced snacks can support a healthy metabolism.

QUICK AND NUTRITIOUS SNACK IDEAS
1. Fresh Fruit and Nut Butter:

Pairing: Slice an apple or banana and pair with a tablespoon of almond or peanut butter.
Nutrient Boost: Add a sprinkle of chia seeds or cinnamon for extra nutrients and flavor.
2. Greek Yogurt with Honey and Nuts:

Protein-Rich: A serving of Greek yogurt topped with a drizzle of honey and a handful of nuts like almonds or walnuts.
Probiotic Benefits: Greek yogurt provides beneficial probiotics for gut health.

3. Veggie Sticks with Hummus:

Crunchy Veggies: Slice carrots, cucumbers, bell peppers, and celery.
Dipping: Serve with a side of hummus for a protein and fiber-rich snack.

4. Whole Grain Crackers with Avocado:

Simple Spread: Spread mashed avocado on whole grain crackers.
Flavor Enhancers: Sprinkle with salt, pepper, and a squeeze of lemon juice.

5. Cottage Cheese and Berries:
Sweet and Savory: Combine a bowl of cottage cheese with fresh berries like strawberries, blueberries, or raspberries.
Texture Variety: Add a handful of nuts or seeds for a crunchy texture.

6. Hard-Boiled Eggs:
Protein Pack: Hard-boil eggs in advance for a quick and easy snack.

Seasoning: Sprinkle with a pinch of salt, pepper, and paprika for flavor.

7. Trail Mix:

Homemade Mix: Combine a mix of nuts, seeds, dried fruit, and a few dark chocolate chips.
Portion Control: Be mindful of portion sizes to avoid overeating.

8. Edamame:

Simple Preparation: Steam edamame and sprinkle with a bit of sea salt.
Protein-Rich: Edamame is a great source of plant-based protein.

9. Rice Cakes with Toppings:

Versatile Base: Use whole grain rice cakes as a base.
Toppings: Add almond butter and banana slices, or cottage cheese and cucumber slices.

10. Popcorn:

Healthy Version: Air-pop popcorn and season with nutritional yeast, a bit of salt, or spices like paprika or cinnamon.
Whole Grain: Popcorn is a whole grain and provides fiber.

DELICIOUS AND NUTRITIOUS SMOOTHIE RECIPES

1. Green Power Smoothie:

Ingredients:
1 cup spinach
1 frozen banana
1/2 cup Greek yogurt
1/2 cup almond milk
1 tablespoon chia seeds
1 tablespoon honey

Instructions:
Blend all ingredients until smooth.
Serve immediately and enjoy a nutrient-packed green smoothie.

2. Berry Blast Smoothie:

Ingredients:
1 cup mixed berries (strawberries, blueberries, raspberries)
1/2 cup Greek yogurt

1/2 cup coconut water
1 tablespoon flaxseeds
1 teaspoon honey (optional)

Instructions:
Blend all ingredients until smooth.
Serve chilled and enjoy the berry goodness.

3. Tropical Mango Smoothie:

Ingredients:
1 cup mango chunks
1/2 cup pineapple chunks
1/2 cup coconut milk
1/2 cup orange juice
1 tablespoon hemp seeds

Instructions:
Blend all ingredients until smooth.
Enjoy a taste of the tropics with this refreshing smoothie.

4. Chocolate Peanut Butter Protein Smoothie:

Ingredients:
1 frozen banana
1 tablespoon peanut butter
1 tablespoon cocoa powder
1 scoop chocolate protein powder
1 cup almond milk

Instructions:
Blend all ingredients until smooth.
Enjoy a rich, protein-packed smoothie.

5. Creamy Avocado Smoothie:

Ingredients:
1/2 avocado
1 frozen banana
1/2 cup spinach
1 cup almond milk
1 tablespoon honey
1 teaspoon vanilla extract

Instructions:
Blend all ingredients until smooth.
Serve immediately for a creamy and nutritious smoothie.

TIPS FOR HEALTHY SNACKING AND SMOOTHIE MAKING

1. Plan and Prepare:

Pre-Portion Snacks: Prepare and portion out snacks ahead of time to grab when you're hungry.
Smoothie Packs: Create smoothie packs by pre-portioning and freezing ingredients for easy blending.

2. Balance Nutrients:

Include Protein: Ensure snacks and smoothies have a source of protein to keep you fuller longer.
Add Fiber: Incorporate fiber-rich foods like fruits, vegetables, and whole grains to aid digestion.

3. Watch Portions:

Moderation: Be mindful of portion sizes to avoid excessive calorie intake.
Listen to Your Body: Eat when you're hungry and stop when you're satisfied.

4. Hydrate:

Drink Water: Complement your snacks and smoothies with plenty of water throughout the day.
Avoid Sugary Drinks: Opt for water, herbal teas, or other low-sugar beverages instead of sugary drinks.

5. Experiment with Flavors:

Try New Recipes: Keep snacking and smoothie-making exciting by trying new recipes and ingredients.
Flavor Combinations: Mix and match different fruits, vegetables, nuts, and seeds to find your favorite combinations.

CONCLUSION
Healthy snacks and smoothies are an excellent way to maintain energy, manage hunger, and ensure you get a variety of nutrients throughout the day. By incorporating a range of nutritious options and following practical tips, you can make smart choices that support your overall health and well-being. Use these recipes and ideas to create satisfying snacks and smoothies that keep you energized and nourished between meals.

SPECIAL OCCASION MEALS: CELEBRATING WITH HEALTH IN MIND
Special occasions are times to celebrate with family and friends, often around a shared meal. While these events are traditionally associated with indulgent foods, it's entirely possible to create delicious and festive dishes that are also healthy. This chapter provides ideas and recipes for special occasion meals that balance indulgence with nutrition, allowing you to enjoy celebrations without compromising your health.

THE IMPORTANCE OF HEALTHY SPECIAL OCCASION MEALS

1. Balanced Indulgence:

Enjoyment without Guilt: Creating healthier versions of traditional dishes allows you to indulge in your favorite foods without feeling guilty.
Nutrient Density: Even on special occasions, it's important to include nutrient-dense foods to support overall health.

2. Maintaining Well-Being:

Energy Levels: Eating balanced meals helps maintain energy levels during busy celebrations.
Digestive Health: Opting for lighter, healthier options can prevent the discomfort often associated with overeating rich, heavy foods.

3. Inclusive Eating:

Accommodating Needs: Healthy special occasion meals can accommodate various dietary needs and preferences, ensuring all guests can enjoy the celebration.
Healthy and Festive Special Occasion Recipes

1. Herb-Crusted Roast Turkey:

Ingredients:
1 whole turkey (10-12 pounds)
1/4 cup olive oil
2 tablespoons fresh rosemary, chopped
2 tablespoons fresh thyme, chopped
2 tablespoons fresh sage, chopped
4 garlic cloves, minced
Salt and pepper to taste

Instructions:
Preheat the oven to 325°F (165°C).
In a small bowl, mix olive oil, herbs, garlic, salt, and pepper.
Rub the herb mixture all over the turkey, including under the skin.
Place the turkey on a roasting rack in a roasting pan.

Roast for approximately 3-4 hours, or until the internal temperature reaches 165°F (74°C).
Let rest for 20 minutes before carving.

2. Quinoa Stuffed Bell Peppers:

Ingredients:
6 bell peppers, tops cut off and seeds removed
1 cup quinoa, cooked
1 cup black beans, drained and rinsed
1 cup corn kernels
1 cup diced tomatoes
1/2 cup shredded cheese (optional)
1 teaspoon cumin
1 teaspoon chili powder
Salt and pepper to taste

Instructions:
Preheat the oven to 375°F (190°C).
In a large bowl, combine cooked quinoa, black beans, corn, tomatoes, cumin, chili powder, salt, and pepper.
Stuff each bell pepper with the quinoa mixture and place in a baking dish.
If using, sprinkle cheese on top of each pepper.
Cover with foil and bake for 30 minutes. Remove foil and bake for an additional 10 minutes.
Serve warm.

3. Balsamic Glazed Salmon:

Ingredients:
4 salmon fillets
1/4 cup balsamic vinegar
2 tablespoons honey
1 tablespoon Dijon mustard
2 garlic cloves, minced
Salt and pepper to taste

Instructions:
Preheat the oven to 400°F (200°C).
In a small bowl, whisk together balsamic vinegar, honey, Dijon mustard, and garlic.
Place salmon fillets on a baking sheet lined with parchment paper.
Brush the balsamic glaze over the salmon fillets.
Bake for 15-20 minutes, or until the salmon is cooked through.
Serve with a side of roasted vegetables or a fresh salad.

4. Cauliflower Mashed Potatoes:

Ingredients:

1 large head cauliflower, cut into florets
2 tablespoons butter
1/4 cup Greek yogurt
2 garlic cloves, minced
Salt and pepper to taste

Instructions:

Steam cauliflower florets until tender.
In a food processor, blend cauliflower, butter, Greek yogurt, and garlic until smooth.
Season with salt and pepper to taste.
Serve as a healthy alternative to traditional mashed potatoes.

5. Mixed Berry Parfait:

Ingredients:

2 cups Greek yogurt
1 cup mixed berries (strawberries, blueberries, raspberries)
1/4 cup granola
1 tablespoon honey
Fresh mint leaves for garnish

Instructions:

In serving glasses, layer Greek yogurt, mixed berries, and granola.
Drizzle with honey.
Garnish with fresh mint leaves.
Serve immediately or refrigerate until ready to serve.

TIPS FOR HEALTHY CELEBRATIONS

1. Focus on Whole Foods:

Fresh Ingredients: Use fresh, whole ingredients to prepare dishes that are both nutritious and flavorful.
Homemade: Opt for homemade recipes to control the ingredients and avoid processed foods.

2. Balance Your Menu:

Variety: Include a variety of dishes that offer a balance of lean proteins, whole grains, and plenty of vegetables.
Portion Control: Serve smaller portions of indulgent dishes alongside larger portions of nutrient-dense foods.

3. Lighten Up Traditional Recipes:

Healthy Swaps: Make healthier versions of traditional recipes by swapping out high-calorie ingredients for lighter alternatives.
Reduce Sugar and Fat: Cut down on sugar and fat without sacrificing flavor by using natural sweeteners and healthy fats.

4. Hydrate:

Water: Encourage drinking water by serving infused water with fresh fruits and herbs.
Limit Alcohol: Offer a variety of non-alcoholic beverages and limit alcohol consumption.

5. Mindful Eating:

Savor Each Bite: Encourage mindful eating by savoring each bite and eating slowly.
Listen to Your Body: Pay attention to hunger and fullness cues to avoid overeating.

6. Stay Active:

Active Traditions: Incorporate physical activities into your celebrations, such as a walk after dinner or a game of frisbee.
Balance with Exercise: Balance indulgent meals with regular physical activity to maintain overall health.

CONCLUSION
Celebrating special occasions with healthy meals allows you to enjoy festive moments without compromising your well-being. By focusing on balanced, nutrient-dense dishes and making mindful choices, you can create memorable and delicious meals that support your health. Use these recipes and tips to plan special occasion meals that are both satisfying and nutritious, ensuring your celebrations are joyful and health-conscious.

MOVING FORWARD

DEVELOPING A HEALTHY RELATIONSHIP WITH FOOD

A healthy relationship with food is essential for overall well-being. It involves understanding and honoring your body's nutritional needs, enjoying a variety of foods without guilt, and cultivating mindful eating practices. This chapter explores strategies for developing a positive and balanced relationship with food that promotes both physical and mental health.

THE IMPORTANCE OF A HEALTHY RELATIONSHIP WITH FOOD

1. Mental Well-Being:

Reduced Anxiety: A balanced approach to eating can reduce anxiety around food choices and eating habits.
Improved Self-Esteem: Feeling confident about your food choices contributes to a positive self-image and higher self-esteem.

2. Physical Health:

Balanced Nutrition: A healthy relationship with food ensures you get a wide range of nutrients essential for bodily functions.
Weight Management: Listening to your body's hunger and fullness cues helps maintain a healthy weight naturally.

3. Emotional Fulfillment:

Enjoyment: Food is a source of pleasure and enjoyment. Embracing this aspect can enhance your overall life satisfaction.
Connection: Sharing meals with others fosters social connections and emotional bonding.

STRATEGIES FOR DEVELOPING A HEALTHY RELATIONSHIP WITH FOOD

1. Embrace Mindful Eating:

Be Present: Focus on your eating experience by eliminating distractions such as TV or smartphones.
Savor Your Food: Take time to savor the flavors, textures, and aromas of your food.
Listen to Your Body: Pay attention to hunger and fullness cues, and eat when you're hungry and stop when you're satisfied.

2. Reject Diet Culture:

Avoid Restrictive Diets: Steer clear of diets that eliminate entire food groups or severely restrict calories.
Focus on Health, Not Weight: Prioritize overall health and well-being over achieving a specific weight or body size.

3. Practice Balance and Moderation:

Allow All Foods: Include a variety of foods in your diet, recognizing that no single food is "good" or "bad."
Portion Control: Enjoy indulgent foods in moderation without guilt or shame.

4. Cultivate Positive Food Experiences:

Experiment with Recipes: Try new recipes and cooking techniques to make mealtime enjoyable and exciting.
Social Eating: Share meals with family and friends to build positive associations with food.

5. Understand Emotional Eating:

Recognize Triggers: Identify emotional triggers that lead to overeating or undereating.
Develop Coping Strategies: Find healthy ways to cope with emotions, such as talking to a friend, engaging in a hobby, or practicing relaxation techniques.

6. Educate Yourself:

Nutritional Knowledge: Learn about the nutritional value of different foods and how they benefit your body.
Cooking Skills: Enhance your cooking skills to prepare nutritious and delicious meals at home.

TIPS FOR MAINTAINING A HEALTHY RELATIONSHIP WITH FOOD

1. Plan Balanced Meals:

Variety: Include a variety of fruits, vegetables, whole grains, proteins, and healthy fats in your meals.
Meal Prep: Plan and prepare meals ahead of time to ensure you have healthy options available.

2. Set Realistic Goals:

Small Steps: Set achievable goals that focus on positive changes, such as incorporating more vegetables into your diet.

Celebrate Progress: Acknowledge and celebrate your progress towards healthier eating habits.

3. Practice Self-Compassion:

Be Kind to Yourself: Avoid negative self-talk and be compassionate towards yourself, especially if you have setbacks.
Learning Experience: View mistakes as learning opportunities rather than failures.

4. Seek Professional Support:

Nutritionist or Dietitian: Consult with a nutritionist or dietitian for personalized guidance and support.
Therapist: Consider therapy if you struggle with emotional eating or disordered eating patterns.

5. Stay Hydrated:

Drink Water: Make water your primary beverage choice to stay hydrated and support overall health.
Limit Sugary Drinks: Reduce consumption of sugary drinks and alcohol.

6. Enjoy Physical Activity:

Find Activities You Love: Engage in physical activities that you enjoy, whether it's dancing, hiking, swimming, or yoga.
Regular Movement: Aim for regular physical activity to support physical and mental well-being.

CONCLUSION

Developing a healthy relationship with food is a lifelong journey that involves understanding your body's needs, practicing mindful eating, and embracing balance and variety. By rejecting diet culture, cultivating positive food experiences, and seeking support when needed, you can build a positive and sustainable approach to eating. Use these strategies to foster a healthy relationship with food, ensuring that it nourishes both your body and your soul.

MINDFUL EATING: LISTENING TO YOUR BODY

Mindful eating is a practice that encourages awareness of the present moment and fosters a deeper connection with food. By paying attention to sensations, thoughts, and emotions while eating, you can cultivate a healthier relationship with food and better respond to your body's nutritional needs. This chapter explores the principles of mindful eating and how to incorporate them into your daily life.

UNDERSTANDING MINDFUL EATING

1. Awareness of Eating Habits:

Present Moment: Mindful eating involves being fully present during meals, focusing on the sensory experience of eating.
Eating Cues: Recognize physical hunger cues versus emotional or environmental triggers for eating.

2. Attentive to Food Choices:

Conscious Choices: Make conscious decisions about what to eat based on nutritional value and personal preferences.
Savoring: Take time to savor and appreciate the flavors, textures, and aromas of food.

3. Recognizing Fullness:

Listening to Signals: Tune into your body's signals of hunger and fullness to avoid overeating or undereating.
Pause and Assess: Pause during meals to assess how hungry or full you feel before continuing to eat.

PRINCIPLES OF MINDFUL EATING

1. Engage Your Senses:

Sight: Notice the colors and presentation of your food.
Smell: Appreciate the aromas before taking a bite.
Touch: Feel the textures of different foods in your mouth.

2. Slow Down:

Chew Thoroughly: Chew each bite slowly and thoroughly to aid digestion and enhance satisfaction.
Pause Between Bites: Put down utensils between bites to focus on enjoying the food and recognizing fullness.

3. Non-Judgmental Awareness:

Acceptance: Approach eating without judgment or guilt about food choices.
Self-Compassion: Be kind to yourself if you notice mindless eating habits or emotional triggers.

4. Appreciate Your Food:

Gratitude: Cultivate gratitude for the nourishment and pleasure that food provides.
Connection: Acknowledge the effort and resources that went into producing and preparing your meals.

PRACTICAL TIPS FOR PRACTICING MINDFUL EATING

1. Start Small:

One Meal at a Time: Begin with one meal per day to practice mindful eating techniques.
Gradual Progress: Over time, incorporate mindful eating into more meals and snacks.

2. Minimize Distractions:

Turn Off Screens: Eat without distractions such as television, smartphones, or computers.
Focus on Eating: Pay attention to the meal and the experience of eating.

3. Portion Control:

Serving Size Awareness: Use smaller plates and bowls to control portion sizes.
Listen to Your Body: Stop eating when you feel comfortably full, even if there is food left on your plate.

4. Meal Preparation:

Plan Ahead: Prepare meals in advance to reduce rushed eating and stress during meal times.
Mindful Cooking: Practice mindfulness while cooking, focusing on ingredients and cooking techniques.

5. Practice Gratitude:

Before Meals: Take a moment to express gratitude for the food and those who contributed to it.
After Meals: Reflect on the nourishment and enjoyment you experienced during the meal.

BENEFITS OF MINDFUL EATING

1. Improved Digestion:

Enhanced Awareness: Better digestion and nutrient absorption from chewing food thoroughly and eating more slowly.
Reduced Discomfort: Minimized digestive discomfort like bloating or indigestion.

2. Weight Management:

Natural Control: Better regulation of appetite and portion sizes, leading to weight maintenance or gradual weight loss.
Decreased Overeating: Reduced tendency to overeat in response to emotional triggers or external cues.

3. Emotional Well-Being:

Reduced Stress: Lower stress levels associated with eating, promoting relaxation and enjoyment.
Emotional Regulation: Improved ability to recognize and manage emotional eating patterns.

INCORPORATING MINDFUL EATING INTO DAILY LIFE

1. Reflect Regularly:

Daily Check-In: Take a few moments each day to reflect on your eating habits and how you felt during meals.
Adjust as Needed: Make adjustments based on your observations to improve your mindful eating practice.

2. Seek Support:

Community or Groups: Join mindfulness or mindful eating groups for support and motivation.
Professional Guidance: Consult with a dietitian or therapist specializing in mindful eating for personalized guidance.

3. Persevere and Adapt:

Be Patient: Mindful eating is a skill that develops over time with practice and patience.
Adapt to Challenges: Adjust your approach as needed to overcome challenges and maintain consistency.

CONCLUSION
Mindful eating offers a holistic approach to nourishing your body and cultivating a positive relationship with food. By practicing awareness, appreciation, and self-compassion during meals, you can enhance your overall well-being and satisfaction with eating. Use the principles and tips in this chapter to incorporate mindful eating into your daily life, promoting health, happiness, and mindful living.

STAYING MOTIVATED AND OVERCOMING CHALLENGES

Maintaining motivation and overcoming challenges are essential aspects of any journey toward better health and well-being. Whether you're striving to eat healthier, exercise more, or adopt mindful eating practices, this chapter explores strategies to stay motivated and navigate obstacles effectively.

UNDERSTANDING MOTIVATION

1. Internal vs. External Motivation:

Internal: Motivation that comes from personal values, goals, and enjoyment of the process.
External: Motivation driven by external rewards or pressures, such as praise or social approval.

2. Sustainable Motivation:

Intrinsic Rewards: Focus on the intrinsic rewards of healthier habits, such as feeling energetic or improving mood.
Goal Alignment: Align goals with your values and long-term aspirations for greater motivation.

STRATEGIES FOR STAYING MOTIVATED

1. Set Clear Goals:

Specific and Achievable: Define clear, realistic goals that are achievable within a specific timeframe.
Break It Down: Divide larger goals into smaller, manageable milestones to track progress.

2. Find Your Why:

Personal Meaning: Identify why improving your health is important to you personally.
Visualize Success: Visualize the benefits of achieving your goals to maintain motivation during challenging times.

3. Celebrate Successes:

Acknowledge Achievements: Celebrate small victories along the way to stay motivated and build momentum.
Reward Yourself: Treat yourself to non-food rewards for reaching milestones.

4. Stay Positive:

Optimistic Outlook: Cultivate a positive mindset and believe in your ability to overcome challenges.
Self-Encouragement: Practice self-affirmations and positive self-talk to boost confidence.

OVERCOMING COMMON CHALLENGES

1. Time Constraints:

Prioritize: Allocate time for healthy habits by scheduling them into your daily routine.
Efficiency: Opt for shorter workouts or prepare quick, nutritious meals ahead of time.

2. Social Pressures:

Communicate Boundaries: Clearly communicate your health goals and boundaries to friends and family.
Seek Support: Surround yourself with supportive individuals who encourage your healthy choices.

3. Emotional Eating:

Awareness: Recognize emotional triggers that lead to overeating or unhealthy food choices.
Healthy Coping Strategies: Develop alternative ways to manage emotions, such as journaling or exercise.

4. Plateaus and Setbacks:

Learn from Setbacks: View setbacks as learning opportunities rather than failures.
Adjust Strategies: Modify your approach, such as trying new exercises or seeking professional guidance.

BUILDING RESILIENCE

1. Persistence: Stay committed to your goals despite setbacks or challenges.

Adaptability: Be flexible and willing to adjust your approach as needed to maintain progress.

2. Support Network:

Accountability: Partner with a friend, family member, or health coach to hold you accountable.
Community: Join groups or forums where you can share experiences and receive encouragement.

3. Self-Care:

Balance: Prioritize self-care practices such as adequate sleep, stress management, and relaxation techniques.
Recharge: Take breaks and engage in activities that rejuvenate your mind and body.

MOTIVATION MAINTENANCE TIPS

1. Track Your Progress:

Keep Records: Use a journal or app to track your achievements, workouts, or meals.
Visualize Improvement: Review your progress regularly to stay motivated and identify areas for improvement.

2. Renew Your Commitment:

Revisit Goals: Reflect on your initial reasons for starting your health journey and reaffirm your commitment.
Set New Challenges: Continuously set new goals to maintain motivation and prevent complacency.

3. Seek Inspiration:

Inspiring Stories: Read success stories or follow individuals who inspire you to stay motivated.
Educate Yourself: Stay informed about health topics and explore new ways to enhance your well-being.

CONCLUSION
Staying motivated and overcoming challenges are integral to achieving and maintaining a healthy lifestyle. By setting clear goals, cultivating intrinsic motivation, and developing resilience, you can navigate obstacles and sustain your progress over time. Use the strategies and tips in this chapter to stay motivated, overcome challenges, and enjoy the journey toward improved health and well-being.

CONCLUSION

In "A Woman's Guide to Nutrition: Fueling Your Body with the Right Foods for Every Stage of Life," we have explored the multifaceted landscape of woman's health and nutrition. From childhood through adolescence, pregnancy, midlife, and beyond, this book has provided comprehensive insights and practical guidance to empower women in making informed decisions about their nutrition.

Throughout these pages, we have emphasized the importance of nurturing a healthy relationship with food, practicing mindful eating, and understanding the diverse nutritional needs that evolve with each life stage. By embracing balanced nutrition, incorporating whole foods, and fostering mindfulness in eating habits, women can optimize their health and well-being.

We have delved into the significance of macronutrients and micronutrients, hydration, and the impact of various dietary choices, including plant-based diets and managing food allergies. Each topic has been approached with the aim of equipping women with the knowledge and tools to make choices that support vitality, energy, and longevity.

Moreover, this book has addressed practical aspects such as meal planning, reading food labels, and navigating social settings and travel while maintaining nutritional goals. By offering recipes, meal ideas, and strategies for overcoming challenges, we aimed to ensure that every woman can enjoy delicious, nourishing meals that enhance rather than compromise her health.

As we conclude, it is essential to recognize that achieving optimal nutrition is not just about what we eat but also about how we approach food. Developing a healthy relationship with food involves mindfulness, self-compassion, and a commitment to lifelong learning about nutrition and well-being.

We hope this guide serves as a valuable resource, empowering you to make choices that prioritize your health and vitality. May you continue on your journey with confidence, embracing the principles of balanced nutrition and mindful eating to lead a life of wellness and fulfillment.

Remember, your health is a journey, and every step you take toward nourishing your body and mind is a step toward a healthier, happier you. Here's to celebrating woman's health and nutrition at every stage of life.

www.ingramcontent.com/pod-product-compliance
Lightning Source LLC
Chambersburg PA
CBHW081525250726
48659CB00009B/2938